GARDENING
–for–
MAXIMUM
N·U·T·R·I·T·I·O·N

JERRY MINNICH

Rodale Press, Emmaus, Pa.

Printed in the United States of America on recycled paper containing a high percentage of de-inked fiber.

Book design by Linda Jacopetti
Illustrations by Jack Crane

Library of Congress Cataloging in Publication Data

Minnich, Jerry.
      Gardening for maximum nutrition.

      Bibliography: p.
      Includes index.
      1. Vegetable gardening. 2. Fruit-culture.
3. Vegetables. 4. Fruit. 5. Nutrition. I. Title.
SB321.M64   1983   635   83-3253
ISBN 0-87857-475-1   hardcover

2 4 6 8 10 9 7 5 3 1   hardcover

Contents

CHAPTER 1

The Quality of Your Food— And What You Can Do about It

Maximum nutritional yield from your garden.

That is what this book is all about. At a time when many of us are seriously concerned about the nutritional quality of the foods in our daily diets, and when many are also growing fruits and vegetables at home, it is surprising that so few of us actually plan and plant our gardens with nutrition foremost in mind.

We take up valuable garden space with vegetables of intrinsically low nutritional value. We fail to choose among varieties of the same fruit or vegetable, even though nutritional differences among varieties can be vast. We neglect to treat our soils with proven methods that can enhance the nutritional value of the crops grown therein. And we harvest and preserve our homegrown foods with only the vaguest idea of vitamin and mineral retention.

The fact is that you can *double the total nutritional yield* of your garden with only minor changes in crop selection, soil treatment, planting and cultivation techniques, and harvesting and preservation methods. It will take no more time, no more work, no more garden space—and the garden foods that supply your dinner table will be twice as nutritious as before.

This book will show you how to accomplish this feat. You will learn how to evaluate the nutritional quality of various fruits and vegetables,

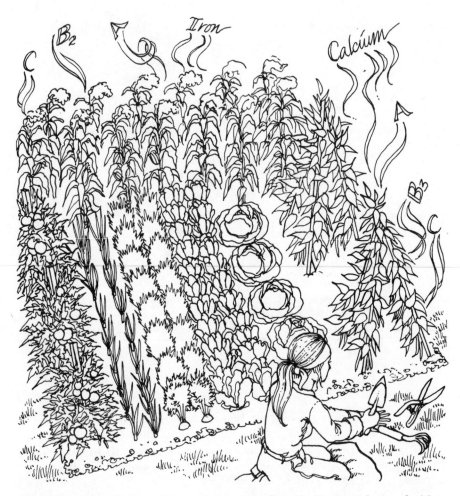

Gold Mine in the Backyard: *You may never actually spot vitamins and minerals rising from the garden, but they're there. Your garden is a valuable source of nutrients with the potential to satisfy most, if not all, of your family's nutritional needs.*

how to build the soil to a point where it can supply crops with optimum amounts of vital nutrients, how to plan and plant your garden to achieve maximum and balanced nutritional yields, and how to preserve that nutritional value through well-conceived and well-executed harvesting and preserving techniques.

In the end, you will never look at your garden in the same way again. You will see it as a major source—perhaps *the* major source—of your family's nutritional needs, a steady supplier of wholesome and high-quality foods. You'll find that your concerns for a good diet and a good garden are, indeed, two sides of the same coin, never again to be considered separately, one without regard to the other.

From now on, you will be gardening for nutrition.

Were Our Grandparents Better Fed?

As a nation, our eating habits have changed drastically over the past 50 years. In our grandparents' time, a typical dinner consisted of meat, potatoes, one or two fresh vegetables, and maybe a hot apple pie. Today, a typical home dinner is more likely to be fried chicken, hash-brown potatoes (both commercially prepared and frozen), and a light salad. In many sections of the country, cooked vegetables never even appear on restaurant menus any more. Our consumption of fresh fruits and vegetables has declined steadily over the years, while that of processed fruits and vegetables has risen sharply.

In the period from 1925 to 1929, Americans ate 168 pounds of fresh potatoes (including sweet potatoes) per person per year. By 1971 (the latest year for which figures are available), that figure had dropped to 62 pounds—a decline of 63 percent. But at the same time, the consumption of processed potatoes (chips, frozen hash-browns, granulated or flaked potatoes, and a myriad of other forms virtually unknown in 1929) had grown to 63 pounds per capita. We now eat more processed than fresh potatoes.

The same trend holds true for other vegetables. From 1925 to 1929, the average American ate 105 pounds of fresh vegetables (not counting potatoes) per year, while in 1971 the total had slipped to 97 pounds. Over

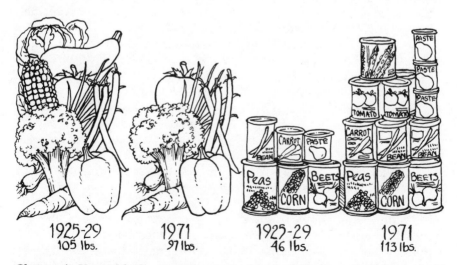

1925-29
105 lbs.

1971
97 lbs.

1925-29
46 lbs.

1971
113 lbs.

Changes in Vegetable Consumption: *In the American diet, the emphasis has gradually shifted toward eating processed rather than fresh vegetables.*

the same period, our per capita consumption of processed vegetables rose from 46 pounds to 113 pounds. We may now be eating more vegetables in total, but more of those are processed rather than fresh vegetables.

Our fruit consumption patterns have been affected largely by the amazing success of the California and Florida citrus fruit industries and particularly by a single product, frozen orange juice, now a staple in most homes. In the past half-century, American consumption of fresh citrus has fallen from 32 to 29 pounds, while that of processed citrus products has gone from virtually nothing to 68 pounds per capita. Total citrus consumption has tripled, and other fruits have suffered from the intense competition. We are now eating only 51 pounds of noncitrus fresh fruit per person. In comparison, our grandparents each ate 109 pounds each year of apples, pears, peaches, berries, and other fruits, many of them grown close to home. The per capita consumption of all noncitrus fruits, both processed and fresh, has declined from 147 to 100 pounds annually, and we are now consuming more citrus than all other kinds of fruit combined.

Once you tally up all these facts and figures, the bottom line is that we are eating 42 percent fewer fresh fruits and vegetables than our grandparents ate (even though distribution methods have improved greatly) and 248 percent more processed fruits and vegetables. What has this change done to the quality of our daily nutrition? There are no simple answers, but several observations may be made.

To start with, any processed food suffers in comparison with the same food in its natural, fresh state. The nutritional quality of the processed food is bound to decline. And since our grandparents ate more fresh and less processed fruits and vegetables, they were better off in this regard. This observation is backed up by solid statistics. According to U.S. government figures, the amount of vitamin A obtained from fruits and vegetables declined from 4,330 International Units per capita between 1925 and 1929 to about 3,860 International Units in 1971—even though total fruit and vegetable consumption increased from 498 to 539 pounds. A little simple arithmetic shows that our fruits and vegetables today are nearly 18 percent lower in vitamin A than those our grandparents enjoyed.

The same is true for other nutrients. Even with the overall increase in consumption, our generation receives 10 percent less thiamine and 20 percent less of both vitamin B_6 and magnesium. It is generally accepted that the nutritional quality of our fruit and vegetable supply is declining.

In all fairness, however, we have improved in some areas. When our grandparents bought fresh fruits and vegetables in the off-season, the quality of those foods was not particularly good. When they were able to find California-grown vegetables at the corner greengrocer, the bedraggled condition of the produce revealed the shortcomings of using ice as the standard means of cooling. Today, refrigerated trucks and railroad cars deliver produce in better condition, although, as we shall see later in this chapter, modern shipping conditions are still far from ideal. There's one point for our generation.

The processed foods that our grandparents ate were likely to be canned, while many fruits and vegetables today are flash-frozen. Strike another point for our generation, since freezing preserves more nutritional quality than canning.

Today, however, many fruits and vegetables are processed into convenience foods that our grandparents never heard of—such delicacies as pop-up fruit tarts for the toaster, dehydrated potatoes for mashing, instant rice (with germ and husk removed), heavily sugared breakfast cereals, pancake mixes, cherry pies at the local fast-food restaurant, and on and on. Rather than preserve a relatively high proportion of vitamins and minerals, as freezing does, these methods decimate nutritional quality. Strike a big one for grandmother.

The fresh fruits and vegetables our grandparents ate were grown much closer to home, and they offered more diversity. Our growing dependence on the citrus industry has deprived us of the variety—in both taste and nutrition—that past generations enjoyed. When we automatically reach for an orange for vitamin C, we miss the vitamin A of a peach or apricot and the trace minerals of an apple or pear. Our grandparents kept nutritional diversity and balance in their diets by depending on local fruits and vegetables in season, for most of the year. Chalk up another point for grandmother.

The last consideration is a dual one, involving the quality of varieties chosen by commercial growers and the quality of the soil in which fruits and vegetables are grown. (More about these later, in chapters 2 and 3.) In short, our current reliance on chemical fertilization and the breeding of food crops without regard for nutrition have joined forces to lower the value of our foods. Once again, grandma comes out ahead.

Adding up all the points for and against, and relying on government figures, the edge would seem to go to the older generation, which ate more fresh produce, grown closer to home, in greater variety, and of generally better quality. If we are to slow this steady erosion of good nutrition and raise the quality of our own diets, we must do it largely on our own, starting in the garden and ending at the dining room table.

How Much Nutrition Can Fruits and Vegetables Give?

Except for the totally self-sufficient gardener who is also a vegetarian, no one's total food supply comes exclusively from the garden. Most of us depend largely on meats, grains, eggs, and dairy products for protein and for a large share of our vitamins and minerals. Still, as recent government figures point out, the fruits and vegetables in our diets provide more than 90 percent of our vitamin C, half of our vitamin A, about a third of the vitamin B_6, a fifth of the thiamine, niacin, and iron, and a fourth of the magnesium. At the same time, fruits and vegetables contribute less than 10 percent of our total calories and a minuscule portion of fat, two things many of us are trying to restrict in our diets.[1]

These, of course, are national averages, and the average diet in America is hardly a laudable one. But you can assure that yours is well above average. By controlling your own daily diet—specifically, by increasing your consumption of low-calorie and low-fat fruits and vegetables and cutting down on heavy meats and processed foods of all kinds—you can increase its overall nutritional quality.

The Quality of Your Food

The quest for high-quality nutrition isn't quite as simple as including certain fruits and vegetables in your diet. Just as important as the *kinds* of foods you choose is the *quality* of those foods. You may know that squash is a good source of vitamin A. But how good is the squash you choose? Is fresh supermarket squash better than commercially frozen squash? You may believe (correctly) that your garden-grown, fresh squash is better than any other, but how does your home-frozen squash compare with fresh supermarket squash? And are certain squash varieties richer in vitamins than others? When it comes to vitamins and minerals in fruits and vegetables, "a rose is a rose is a rose" does not apply. There are serious choices to be made.

The quality of our diets has increasingly come to depend on the quality of foods that others supply to us. In most sections of the country, when winter rolls around, gardeners depend on the local supermarket for their fresh fruits and vegetables. And the proliferation of two-income households has caused many families to depend more and more on restaurant and carry-out meals and on processed and convenience foods for quick home preparation. It is more important than ever that we know something about the way these foods are grown, harvested, processed, and shipped to the supermarket so that we can make the best choice, from a nutritional standpoint, about the foods we eat.

How Much Nutrition in Processed Foods?

We have seen that, as a nation, we are consuming more processed foods and fewer fresh foods with each succeeding generation. How has the change in consumption patterns affected the quality of our diets? No one would reasonably argue that the change has been for the better—but still, we don't know how much worse it is.

Processing invariably destroys some vitamins and minerals, creates nutritional imbalances in others, and involves chemical additives that we would rather not have in our foods. In some cases, processing changes the character of the food so profoundly that it barely resembles its former self. If you ask your child what he had for hot lunch at school, and he claims he doesn't know *what* that stuff was—chances are he isn't kidding.

Take one example, fresh versus processed potatoes. A medium-sized baked potato contains 31 milligrams of vitamin C, while a cup of prepared dehydrated mashed potatoes, weighing the same, has only 5.5 milligrams—meaning that 82 percent of the vitamin C was lost during processing. And if processed foods are "enriched" with vitamin C by the manufacturer in an effort to restore some of the nutrients that have been removed, the laboratory ascorbic acid (pure vitamin C) will not contain the bioflavonoids and other secondary nutrients or companions that enable the body to use vitamin C most effectively. The same principle holds true for other forms of artificial enrichment. A baked potato contains 41 percent more niacin (a member of the vitamin B complex) than does its dehydrated and prepared counterpart. But if the dehydrated potatoes are enriched with laboratory niacin or with one or more of the other recognized B

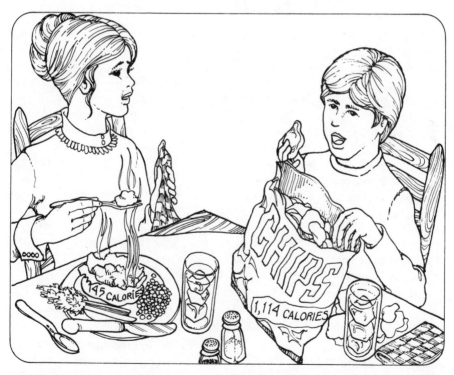

Low Fat vs. High Fat: *That bag of potato chips contains roughly 400 times as much fat as that unadorned baked potato. Processing quickly turns the low-fat, low-calorie potato into a nutritional disaster.*

vitamins, the potatoes still will be missing other components of the B complex that work in concert to serve human nutritional needs.

Processing can not only take away certain elements, it can also add certain elements to foods—and these are usually sugar, fat, and calories. Here's a graphic example. A baked potato is a naturally low-fat food. But when it's processed into dehydrated mashed potatoes, the final product is *23 times higher* in fat content. And if you want an extreme example, consider that an equal amount of potato chips has *400 times as much fat* as that baked potato and contains 1,114 calories versus 145 for the unprocessed potato. In the minds of people who are watching their waistlines, the potato's image has been tarnished by its association with processed junk food. It seems that we've forgotten that the unadorned and unviolated potato is actually a fairly low-calorie vegetable. It's the processing that jacks up the calorie count—and it is processed foods to which, paradoxically, we are turning more and more.

The Quality of "Fresh" Fruits and Vegetables

Nutritional quality is lost not only during processing but also during the growing and delivery of fresh fruits and vegetables to supermarkets and other retail outlets. Nutrients are lost during storage, shipping, and handling, due in part to unfavorable temperature and humidity conditions between the growing fields and the supermarket bin.

The loss in quality begins long before vegetables are even planted in the ground, for the varieties grown commercially are bred not for their nutritional goodness, or even for their taste and texture, but for their ability to withstand abuse. The prime example is the supermarket tomato, which even the least nutrition-conscious shopper knows bears little resemblance to the homegrown variety. Tomato varieties for market growing are, in fact, selected not for their luscious flavor or maximum vitamin C content, but for their ability to drop to the floor without cracking or splitting. The result is a tough-skinned, pale, grainy textured and virtually tasteless fruit which is—to add a final indignity—usually coated with paraffin before it leaves the grower's packing shed.

Traveling with a Pepper

Fresh fruits and vegetables, unlike cheese, bread, and other perishables, are living things. They continue to respire, even after harvest. Chemical changes and enzyme actions continue to alter their character right up to the dinner table. And because they are living things, fresh fruits and vegetables are more susceptible than other perishables to injury and to subsequent loss of nutritional quality.

Let's follow a green pepper from the growing fields of California to the living room of a Cleveland suburb, where it is destined to end up on a fresh-vegetable platter accompanied by a cream-cheese dip.

The first shock for the pepper comes during harvesting. In years past, vegetables were harvested largely by hand, and although the pickers weren't particularly gentle in their handling, they could not match the trauma inflicted by modern mechanical harvesters. These machines dig or pull up the plant, shake it to separate the fruit from the vine, and then roll or drop the fruit into a field cart, hopper, or truck to be driven to the packing shed.

At the shed, the peppers should be cooled to 45° to 50°F to slow down the respiration rate. If they are not, vitamin C quality begins to deteriorate immediately and quickly. The peppers are then graded and sorted, which involves more handling and bruising. On high-speed conveyor belts they are bounced and rolled around, run through cleansing baths, and usually sprayed with a thin layer of paraffin (which, incidentally, has shown carcinogenic action). The wax coating helps to hide bruising and retain moisture in the fruit during the trip east.

Next, the peppers are packed in pallets or crates and sent off to wholesale or retail markets. Not too many years ago, they were packed in small wooden crates, and the top layer of fruit was arranged artfully by hand to appeal to the buyer at auction. Today, most fruits and vegetables are sold not at auction, but sight unseen, usually to buyers for large chain supermarkets. The growers, therefore, have little interest in packing in small crates or in worrying about the eye appeal of the fruit. They may use large pallets, sometimes packing the fruit as tightly as possible by using a vibrating or jiggling device, which causes further bruising and vitamin loss.

The retailer usually receives the peppers in smaller crates made of waxed cardboard, and this requires repacking the fruit at some point along the trip. It is sometimes done at the grower's shed but more often at some midway point—in this case, perhaps in Chicago or even in Cleveland. The repacking involves more rough handling, more exposure to unsuitable temperatures, and further loss of nutritional quality.

Today, truck transportation has replaced rail shipping for the most part, creating more problems for the pepper in its journey. Temperature is critical for maintaining quality of fruits and vegetables. The truck trailer must be refrigerated, and the refrigeration system must be efficient. In too many cases, however, it is far from efficient. The grower or wholesaler may pack the truck too tightly, thus impeding the flow of cool air and preventing it from reaching the center of the load. For transporting frozen foods or cheese, the product is simply loaded in a prechilled state, and then all that is required is running cold air around the perimeter of the load to prevent warm air from entering. But fruits and vegetables respire en route, producing heat. In the trailer, peppers on the perimeter may come close to freezing, while those in the center deteriorate from overheating.

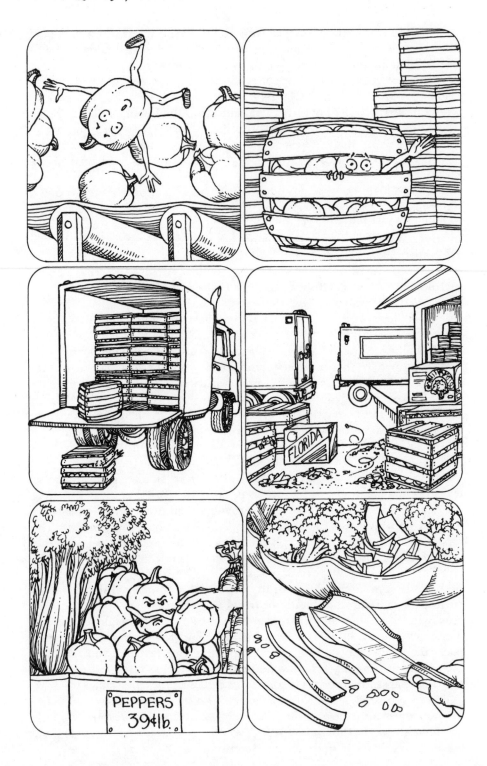

When the peppers finally reach the terminal market, after two thousand miles of bumping and bruising along the highway, a new challenge is presented. They might be shifted to a warehouse or to refrigerated railroad cars and stored until they are needed by the wholesaler. More time passes, with more handling, more bruising, and more temperature and humidity variations. Quality continues to plummet.

After they reach the wholesaler's market, conditions generally become worse. Anyone who has visited these huge produce markets has undoubtedly been appalled to see thousands of crates of fruits and vegetables stacked outside on dirty sidewalks while the exhaust of hundreds of trucks filled the area with carbon monoxide. If it happened to be a hot summer day, so much the worse. Often, shipments are split, opened up and divided into smaller units, causing further damage.

The trip from the terminal market to the supermarket is often a rough one, with the same truck hauling an assortment of fruits and vegetables, each of which has its own temperature requirements. The peppers, which need a range of 45° to 50°F, may be shipped with lettuce, which requires 32°F, and perhaps also with bananas, which need 56° to 60°F. The truck driver may strive for a compromise temperature setting. More often, if the trip is only a few hours long, the driver will not bother at all. The idea is to get the produce to the store before it becomes unsalable. After that, it's the produce manager's problem.

At the supermarket, the peppers may lie around in the storeroom—perhaps refrigerated, perhaps not—until they are needed in the bins in the produce department. Here they undergo further handling by clerks and customers, and are exposed to another range of temperatures. Most produce bins in supermarkets are grossly inefficient, which is why you often seen the produce manager dump shaved ice over the produce or spray it with cold water. Some managers don't even bother to do this much if the fruits and vegetables are moving fast enough. Again, the goal is to get the produce out of the store before it becomes unsalable.

Our particular pepper is examined by the suburban Cleveland host (that wax coating has it looking presentable), tossed into a shopping cart, pushed to the cash register, and stuffed into a grocery bag (but not before the cashier places it gently into its own little plastic bag, as visible evidence of the care with which it is handled). Our host puts the grocery bag into his car and drives home directly—if he doesn't stop for an hour to pay some bills, pick up the wine, or get a haircut. If it's summer, the pepper can be

Traveling with a Pepper: *After being harvested by machine and bounced along a conveyor belt, the jostled pepper comes to rest in the cramped quarters of a shipping crate. A truck hauls the crates of peppers across the country to a wholesalers' market. From there, the none-too-fresh pepper eventually winds up in a produce bin at the local supermarket. After a trip home in a shopping bag, the pepper ends up on a party platter of sliced raw vegetables and dip.*

devastated quickly by the heat. In winter, freezing is a definite possibility. Quality continues to decline.

At home, by the time the pepper hits the vegetable crisper it may have lost half or more of its original vitamin C content along with lesser amounts of other vitamins.

Several hours before the party, the pepper is carefully prepared. The host cuts it into strips, exposing the inner flesh to oxygen and leading to further and rapid loss of vitamin C. And as the clock ticks down to party time, the pepper strips—now without the protection of the skin—continue to lose vitamin C at a very high rate. At eight o'clock, what nutrients remain are consumed amid scintillating party conversation.

The point of this story is not to convince you to stop buying supermarket produce (after all, a beat-up pepper is better than no pepper at all if you're dying for a pepper), but to stress that "fresh" commercial produce is usually not fresh at all. In wintertime, most shoppers would be better off buying frozen vegetables whenever they are available since these will have retained a greater proportion of nutrients than their "fresh" counterparts, which have undergone a long and debilitating journey across the country.

Fortunately, there are other sources of fruits and vegetables besides the supermarket. Much better than the processed, fresh or frozen fruits and vegetables you find there is fresh produce purchased directly from the grower, from roadside stands, or from one of the farmers' markets which are springing up in all parts of the country. When you buy from a farmers' market, it's best to get to know the grower on a personal basis. Strike up a conversation. Ask which variety of broccoli this is, why this particular variety was chosen, what kinds of fertilizer were used, and—especially—when was the crop harvested? You will soon know if this is the grower you are talking to or someone who just brought up a load of produce from the nearest wholesale market. Many farmers' markets insist that produce be locally grown and have restrictions to prevent the sale of produce trucked in from across the country, but it pays to make sure. (If you buy at a farmers' market, consider buying in bulk and then rushing home to freeze all you can. Your nutritional gains will be significant, as will your cash savings.)

Although a farmers' market or roadside stand is a giant step above the local supermarket, there's an even better source of fruits and vegetables— your garden.

Nutritional Potential
of the Home Garden

How much of your family's nutritional needs can be filled directly from your garden? It depends on a number of factors, namely: the size of your garden; the size of your family; how you define *nutritional needs*; the section of the country in which you live and the length of the growing season; and how you go about choosing crops and growing them.

Because all these factors vary from family to family, there's no definitive answer to the question. A family of four, working a 30 by 30-foot garden in a 130-day growing season, can raise enough vegetables to supply nearly all their needs the year round. By using intensive methods, combining short- and long-season crops, and giving emphasis to vegetables for freezing, this modest plot can supply most of their vitamin A and C, nearly one-half of their vitamin B complex and iron, and varying amounts of other vitamins and minerals. By including high-protein crops, they can harvest up to a fourth of their protein needs from this plot—more, if they depend solely on vegetarian protein sources and want to slant their crop selections in this direction. Add some permanent fruit plantings and their overall nutrient totals will be higher.

This example highlights the point that you can double the nutritional yield of your garden, no matter what its size, by using the methods explained in these pages. And because you will be substituting your own garden produce for commercially prepared foods, whether fresh or processed, you will raise your nutritional level to new heights.

Planning Makes a Difference

When you make the decision to garden for nutrition, you'll find yourself spending more time than ever before *planning*. Much as the manager of a retail store considers the income productivity of every square foot of floor space, you will give careful consideration to the nutritional productivity of every foot of garden space. Never fear—this won't take the fun out of gardening. In fact, it will add to it. Planning is a most pleasant activity for those long dark days of January and February, when the seed catalogs arrive to help relieve the winter blahs.

The important things you should plan for are nutritional quality, quantity, and balance. If you took a nutritional survey of last season's garden, you might be surprised to find that certain nutritional elements were grossly underrepresented. Your vegetable crop mix may have yielded ample amounts of vitamins A and C but precious little of the B complex. Your total yield may have been fairly good in calcium content but low in iron. The total protein yield may have been dismal. The reason your garden didn't measure up, of course, is that you didn't plant with nutrition in mind.

If your garden did turn out to be a poor nutritional yielder, you can take some comfort in the realization that you are not alone. A few years ago, a University of California researcher rated 39 common fruits and vegetables according to their total nutritional quality, then compared his rankings with those fruits and vegetables most popular in home gardens.[2] Not surprisingly, he found very little correlation between nutritional goodness and popularity. Of the 10 most nutritious vegetables, only 2 (carrots and sweet potatoes) were also in the top 10 of the popularity rankings. Some of the most nutritious vegetables were also some of the least grown. (To relieve your suspense, here are the scientist's rankings of the most nutritious vegetables, in descending order: broccoli, spinach, Brussels sprouts, lima beans, peas, asparagus, globe artichokes, cauliflower, sweet potatoes, and carrots.)

This year, the nutrient quality of your harvest will be greatly enhanced because you'll be more knowledgeable about choosing both among vegetable crops and among varieties within the same crop. You may decide, for instance, to plant half as much leaf lettuce as before and fill in that free space with spinach. Both produce good springtime salads, but the spinach is 120 percent richer in iron. By tossing a salad that's half lettuce and half spinach, therefore, you'll increase that salad's iron content by 60 percent, a nifty nutritional gain that involves no extra effort or space and no sacrifice in eating pleasure. (Chapter 5 will show you what other kinds of crop substitutions you can make for nutritional gains.)

In choosing among different varieties of the same crop, you should look for nutritional differences, which are sometimes enormous. If you've traditionally planted Table Queen acorn squash, you might consider substituting Jersey Golden Acorn, a 1982 All-American selection that equals Table Queen in taste and texture but contains three times as much vitamin A. When modern fruits and vegetables are supplying 18 percent less vitamin A than those of our grandparents' time, here's an opportunity for us to catch up in a hurry—simply by taking the time to search out and grow nutritionally superior varieties. (Profiles of some superior varieties are given in chapter 2.)

In addition to choosing crops for high nutritional yield and balance, you should pay attention to the quantity of crops which your garden can support. If your garden space is unlimited, of course, getting the most out of every square inch may not be a high priority. But if, like may gardeners, your space is limited, you will be amazed to find that you can greatly increase yields by using intercropping, succession planting, wide-row and double-row planting, and other intensive gardening techniques. All are discussed later, in chapter 5.

While intensive gardening techniques can increase garden yields in terms of space, extending the growing season can increase them in terms of time. By the wise use of cold frames and hotbeds and through other season-extending techniques, you can start garden plants earlier in the spring and extend the autumn harvest period, too. And although space- and time-extending methods are not a major focus of this book (the information is readily available in other books), they are definitely factors to consider when you plan the garden for maximum nutritional yield.

The last major factor to consider in planning is the quality of your garden soil. There is little doubt, despite some lingering claims to the contrary, that what is in your soil has a lot to do with what is in your food. If selenium is deficient in soils, it will be deficient in the foods grown in those soils. If the soil lacks iodine, so will the food that soil produces. Later on, in chapter 3, careful consideration will be given to the often complex relationship between soil quality and food quality—a most important factor in nutritional garden planning.

One final note about the nutrition information in this book. Unless otherwise indicated, all nutritional analysis figures in this book are taken from *Nutritive Value of American Foods in Common Units,* United States Department of Agriculture (USDA), Agriculture Handbook No. 456. Be aware that nutritional analyses vary from test to test, often considerably. However, USDA figures are the most comprehensive available and are used to assure consistent bases of comparison among different foods.

Also keep in mind that this book is primarily a *gardening* book, not a treatise on nutrition. The intent of the author is to tell you, in general terms using general figures as guidelines, what sort of nutritional yield it is possible to harvest from the garden and how you can influence that yield for the better. Now, on to chapter 2 where you'll find out which crops and, specifically, which varieties will provide you with the best nutritional yield.

CHAPTER 2

Advances in High-Nutrition Crops

Although the scientific community has the ability to breed food crops of outstanding nutritional quality, it has never done so except in a limited and sporadic way. The varieties of fruits and vegetables offered today are no better—and in some instances are worse—than those of several generations ago.

Genetic engineering in plant breeding is a highly tuned and sophisticated science. More than at any other time in our history, scientists are able to develop food crop varieties with all the characteristics desired.

The critical questions are: *which* characteristics are desired, and *by whom?* Technological capability is not the problem here. The problem is the national food marketing structure (dominated by economic considerations) that determines which crop characteristics are to be sought and developed in new food crops. And the results of those choices are not necessarily beneficial to those of us who ultimately consume the food.

The first thing to understand is that crop breeding is carried out by public and private universities and by private laboratories for the benefit of agribusiness. When you find numerous seed catalogs flooding the mailbox each January you may gain the impression that plant breeding is carried out for the benefit of home gardeners. After all, dozens of new varieties are introduced each year. But in fact, the home garden market is a minor segment of the seed and plant industry, the major clients being the commercial crop growers who feed more than 200 million Americans and countless others throughout the world. In the face of the enormous economic demands of commercial growers, it is little wonder that the home gardener is a secondary consideration. Many of the new varieties offered in seed catalogs are, in fact, by-products of commercial breeding efforts or are the same new varieties developed for commercial growing. It was not the home gardener who asked for hybrid tomato varieties that produce all their fruit within a two-week span, but the commercial grower who finds it more efficient and profitable to make a single harvest during the growing season.

Because commercial growers and home gardeners have such different priorities, the crop characteristics demanded by one are not necessarily the same as those desired by the other. Commercial crops tend to be bred for size, shape, color, general appearance, uniform time of ripening, ease of harvest, ability to stand up to rough handling and long-term shipping, and—above all—maximum yield. Taste is a factor although a minor one, as evidenced by the typical supermarket tomato. Nutritional quality is rarely a factor at all.

Despite the low status of nutritional quality, plant breeders in recent years have been increasing efforts to develop more nutritious varieties of some crops for home production. But where the really serious crop breeding goes on—for commercial production—the attitude still seems to be that the consumer doesn't care whether a cucumber has 2 milligrams of vitamin C or 200, as long as it looks green and feels firm. Commercial breeders are more interested in developing a square tomato that will reduce shipping space by 34 percent than they are in enhancing the nutritional profile of commercial tomatoes.

Some exceptionally vitamin-rich varieties have been developed quite by accident as researchers sought to develop more attractive color. Few of these varieties have been embraced by the consumer at the supermarket, however, a result not only of nutritional ignorance among consumers, but also of a total lack of consumer education. If a high-vitamin A squash were to be test marketed, what mechanism would there be to inform the shopper of its vitamin content? The fresh fruits and vegetables you find in the produce bins are not labeled, even as to variety.

The fact remains that the genetic engineers, the scientists who breed new crops, are working for the commercial growers. The commercial growers are in business to make maximum profits. And sadly enough, the nutritional quality of foods contributes in no way to profits.

In 1972, the American Medical Association Council on Foods and Nutrition and the United States Department of Agriculture (USDA) sponsored a symposium on nutrition. The papers of that symposium were collected into a volume, *Nutritional Qualities of Fresh Fruits and Vegetables.* Among the papers, many of which held some very valuable information, was one by Edwin A. Crosby, Ph.D., director of the Agriculture Division of the National Canners Association. In it, Dr. Crosby gives his reasons why nutrition does not play a part in plant breeding and, indeed, why it should not play a part. Here are some salient excerpts from that paper:

Let us look at why fruits and vegetables are included in the American diet. It seems there are two basic reasons, one nutritional and the other esthetic. From the standpoint of nutrition, principal consideration given to fresh fruits and vegetables should be in the area of vitamin content and, secondarily, mineral content. It is to be questioned, however, whether the average housewife thinks about nutrition when she buys these products or whether she isn't more concerned about variety, color, esthetics, flavor, texture and other factors in her menu planning. If we move to nutritional labeling, we may well have a large number of consumers awakened to the realization that fruits and vegetables are not generally good sources of nutrients from an economic standpoint, and if consumers are truly concerned about insuring that their families receive enough vitamins and minerals, the easy, economical route to insure this end is to purchase them in pill form. It would indeed be difficult strictly on an economic basis to justify the purchase of fruits and vegetables for their nutritional values because the nutrients they contain can be better obtained, in terms of cost, from other sources. If tomorrow's housewife becomes a nutritional bug with a calculator in her pocket when she goes to the supermarket and thinks only of value in terms of nutrition, she will avoid the purchase of fruits and vegetables.

It is evident that through genetic engineering, improved cultural techniques, and careful attention to storage and marketing practices, the nutritional qualities of fruits and vegetables can be improved. The real question, however, is whether improved nutritional value for fresh fruits and vegetables is truly important to the public welfare. Should this area of research be given priority or should we look to vitamin pills or fortified processed products as may be desirable to improve nutrition? What choices will the consumer make if we move to nutritional labeling of fresh fruits and vegetables as well as processed foods? If higher nutritional values in these products mean higher costs, the decision of the economy-minded buyer is obvious. A simple pill can well be a preferable alternative to paying for higher nutritional values in fresh fruits and vegetables.

It is important to recognize priorities in meeting the need for total food production. Priorities in respect to the production of fruits and vegetables must include the factors which keep our agriculture competitive in domestic and world markets. It is only logical that emphasis be placed on factors such as yield; harvestability; storage, shipping and handling qualities; color, flavor, and general consumer acceptance; disease and insect resistance. When it comes to the economics of genetic engineering, these factors have been given preference in the past and should continue to be given emphasis in the future. The battle for survival in agriculture will continue and it will not be helped by a redirection of emphasis in breeding and development of new varieties toward nutritional quality improvement.

In spite of the possibilities and promise of doing certain things through genetic engineering to improve the nutritional values of our fruits and vegetables, where are the economic reasons justifying such efforts?[1]

So much for the hope of getting more nutritious fruits and vegetables through the efforts of crop scientists. Now let's take a very brief look at the attitudes of the commercial growers. In our grandparents' time, the family farmer raised maximum yields of crops by attempting to be a good farmer. He knew that the land was his life and that his income depended to a large extent on how well he treated the soil. Granted, American farmers of earlier times adopted some terrible agronomic practices, some of which led to the dust-bowl conditions of the 1930s. There is no point in being overly romantic about it. Still, at least until after World War II, there was a strong tradition of the family farm in America, the sense that this farm would be passed down from generation to generation. The farmer had a sense of pride as he looked out over a field—*his* field—of new spring crops emerging from the soil.

Today, fewer and fewer crops are being raised by farmers on their own land. More crops are being raised on fewer and larger farms, and nearly all of the growing is being done by hired hands while the owners sit in corporate offices hundreds or thousands of miles away. Farming has become less a way of life and more a process of large-scale food manufacturing. An example—perhaps extreme, but by no means unusual today—is related by Ross Hume Hall, Ph.D., professor of biochemistry at McMaster University, in the *Journal of Holistic Medicine:*

Roy Berry, a farmer near Hamilton, Ontario, sold his 125-acre farm to a land speculator in 1972. The Berry family continued living in the farmhouse on their former land. The land speculator, for the past eight years, has leased the farm to York Canners, a large, diversified agri-business that operates hundreds of similar leased farms, on which it produces vegetables destined for canning.

The Berry farm lies on gently rolling land. In spring, as it dries out from winter snow, the higher portions are ready for working sooner than the lower, more soggy parts. During the years that Mr. Berry farmed the land, he watched the weather closely, ploughing and preparing the ground as it became ready. Now, at no particular

> *time in spring, flatbed trucks arrive, discharging equipment and men.*
> *Within 2 to 3 hours, the entire farm has been tilled, planted,*
> *fertilized, and deweeded with a herbicide. The equipment and crew*
> *then disappear, not to be seen again until harvest time. The crop,*
> *usually corn, never ripens evenly. Nevertheless, at some instant, day*
> *or night in harvest season, trucks laden with heavy equipment roll in*
> *and within a short time the entire crop, ready or not, has been*
> *harvested.*[2]

So much for the hope of getting better-quality fruits and vegetables through the efforts of the commercial growers. And it's probably hopeless to count on the efforts of the supermarket produce manager, as well. So where does that leave us?

It leaves us in the garden, that's where. In order to get high-quality fruits and vegetables rich in vitamins and minerals, we must adopt wise soil-treatment practices, proper cultural and harvesting techniques, and good storage and cooking methods. And above and beyond all that, we must seek out and find those varieties of food crops that have, through accident or design, been bred to contain higher than average levels of the essential vitamins and minerals.

Today, there are relatively few of these varieties around. In this chapter, current knowledge is summarized so that you can take advantage of these select crops in your own garden plan. But the only way you will see more of these varieties in the future is through constant demand and increasing public pressure. If home gardeners make it a point to buy nutritionally superior varieties, this will create a demand and thus encourage the development of similar varieties of other crops. In the political realm, you can take action by encouraging your congressional representatives and officials at the USDA to increase research efforts in this area.

Another important step is to press for nutritional labeling not only on processed fruits and vegetables, but on fresh ones, as well. That way, nutrition-conscious shoppers would know what variety of broccoli is in the supermarket produce bin and what its average vitamin C content is. If carrots were labeled as to their vitamin A content, perhaps consumers would soon begin to pay attention to the nutritional differences among varieties. If the protein quality of supermarket potatoes has been slipping in the past several decades (and there is evidence to support the belief that it has), how is the consumer to know except by forcing the grower to label the potatoes and by having the USDA make periodic checks on those potatoes to ensure the accuracy of the labels? It is certainly not the aim of this book to foment political action. Nevertheless, when it comes to nutritional quality and the resultant health and well-being of the general public, it is not too much to expect the government to take a role in seeing that people are informed about the foods they buy, much as it has taken a

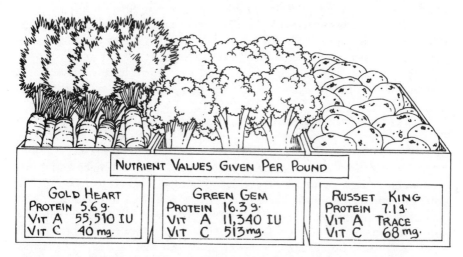

Signs for Nutrition-Conscious Shoppers: *Many frozen and canned goods list nutritional data, but when it comes to fresh produce the consumer doesn't have much to go on. Perhaps someday, in the not too distant future, produce sections will feature helpful signs such as these to guide your purchasing.*

role in other areas of consumer information. Certainly the job will not be taken up voluntarily by the agribusiness sector.

Superior Vegetables and Fruits

This section gives you a brief look at some crops and crop varieties that have, in various ways, proved to be superior in vitamin or mineral content. Try to work as many of these crops as you can into the garden plan, and you will enhance the nutritional quality of your harvest considerably. You will also demonstrate, to the seed houses, at least, that you do indeed care about the nutritional quality of the foods you grow. And by making that simple statement, perhaps you will contribute to the development of more such varieties in the years ahead. (For a listing of seed houses that carry these particular crops, see Seed Sources for Superior Vegetables and Fruits and Seed Sources Directory in the appendix.)

Amaranth

Amaranth is the most nutritious vegetable you can grow in your garden. It is an exceptionally rich source of calcium, iron, and vitamin C; a very rich source of potassium, vitamin A, and riboflavin; a rich source of niacin; and an above-average source of protein. As a nutritional package, among all garden crops, it is approached only by sunflower seeds.

There are two kinds of amaranth—grain and vegetable. Since grain amaranth is suitable mainly for large-scale production and not for home gardens, all references to amaranth in this book are to the vegetable type, a quickly growing annual that can be used like spinach, raw in salads or steamed as a potherb. Amaranth leaves also make a savory addition to soups and stews.

It's difficult to overstress amaranth's potential contribution to the diet. This leafy green is the richest of all vegetables in calcium, having nearly twice the content of its nearest competitor, collards. No other vegetable is higher in iron; amaranth has more than twice the iron of spinach and much more per serving than dry beans, which are noted for their iron content. In potassium, it ranks among the top ten fruits and vegetables, along with soybeans. Amaranth is also in the top ten in vitamin A content, ranking between spinach and butternut squash. In terms of riboflavin, it ranks with turnip and dandelion greens, both rich sources. Amaranth has the distinction of being the only green, leafy vegetable to rank in the top ten in niacin content. And in vitamin C, it is exceeded only by broccoli, ranking far ahead of such noteworthy crops as sweet peppers, kale, collards, muskmelons, and strawberries. Amaranth even stands up well when compared with citrus fruits; 4 ounces of amaranth contain as much vitamin C as 6 ounces of orange juice.

Although amaranth has been grown for human food for more than four thousand years, it has only recently received renewed attention as a crop for North American gardens. This is one leafy green that does best in hot weather, making it a good succession crop to follow spinach. Amaranth has been too long neglected and deserves a spot in every garden.

Adzuki Bean

Adzuki beans are a Japanese import Americans can be grateful for. In Japan, these small, maroon beans are extremely popular. They're made into a sweetened paste that goes into everything from soups and pastries to Popsicles and soft drinks. Initial reports on the adzuki indicated that its protein content and quality were far superior to any other bean. Although these first reports were somewhat exaggerated, tests have now confirmed that the adzuki is certainly on a par with soybeans in protein content, containing about 25 percent protein of a very high quality.

Adzuki beans are easier to use than soybeans in their dry form since they cook up in a short time. Their taste is excellent—nutty and sweet— qualifying them as a good vegetable dish by themselves or served on a bed of rice. Adzuki beans will certainly grow in popularity as their qualities become better known in the Western world.

Imperator Carrot

In 1928, the Asgrow Seed Company developed a long, tapering carrot that was not brittle and did not break easily during transportation. It also had an attractive, deep orange color. The company had, in other words, developed an ideal market carrot. Quite by accident, the new Imperator carrot was also far richer in vitamin A than other carrots. This was precisely because of its deep orange color, produced by its very high carotene content. Carotene, of course, provides provitamin A, which is converted into true vitamin A by the human body. From that time until the present, Imperator has been a favorite market carrot.

You can easily judge the vitamin A content of carrots (as well as squash, muskmelons, peaches, and other orange-fleshed vegetables and fruits) by the deepness of their orange color. As a general guideline, the deeper the orange, the higher the carotene content, and the more vitamin A there will be. You can also judge the vitamin A content during various stages of growth since the concentration of carotene increases as the fruits or roots grow to maturity.

Superior Apple Varieties

Although apples are not a significant source of vitamin C, there are some varieties that are richer in this vitamin than others. The USDA figures for vitamin C content of apples are based on a sampling of the most important commercial varieties—Delicious, Golden Delicious, McIntosh, and Rome. On this basis, the average vitamin C content was found to be 6 milligrams in one medium-size (5⅓ ounces) apple. However, there is a wide variation in vitamin C content among apple varieties.[3] This list of 11 apple varieties, in descending order of vitamin C content, will help you choose from the varieties highest in this vitamin when planting trees at home.

Apple Variety	Milligrams Vitamin C in 5⅓ ounces
Wegener	29
Northern Spy	24
Rome Beauty	17
Golden Delicious	15
Jubilee	15
Winesap	14
Jonathan	11
Delicious (red)	9
Stayman	9
Spartan	5
McIntosh	3

Orlando Gold Carrot

A new hybrid carrot, developed by USDA experiment stations in Florida, Wisconsin, Texas, California, Arizona, and Idaho, is reported to be 50 percent higher in vitamin A than Imperator. Orlando Gold was not yet on the market as of this writing but will be offered to the general public first by Northrup King. Since you can't buy seeds directly from Northrup King, watch for their seed packets to appear in racks in the local garden center.

Early Snowball Cauliflower

When choosing among cauliflower varieties, consider Early Snowball, a 1941 introduction of the Ferry Morse Seed Company. Early Snowball, as its name indicates, is an early maturer (50 to 60 days), has good quality and flavor, and most important of all, contains more vitamin C than other popular varieties. It is also rich in potassium and calcium and offers fairly good amounts of vitamin A and some of the B-complex vitamins. Remember that the tender leaves cradling the flower head are far richer in vitamin C than the head itself and should not be trimmed off as a matter of course when you prepare the vegetable for the table. (This is true of all cauliflower varieties and of broccoli, as well.) Retain some of the leaves, which have a taste resembling Brussels sprouts, and get into the habit of eating them along with the florets. When you do, every serving of cauliflower will offer a nutritional bonus, no matter what the variety.

Dwarf Scotch Kale

For such a humble-looking crop, kale packs a nutritional wallop. It's a very rich source of vitamin C, ranking fifth among all garden crops; a rich source of calcium, ranking seventh in this category; and a good source of vitamin A, riboflavin, and niacin. And of all the kales, Dwarf Scotch is the most nutritious. It's best eaten raw for peak nutritional value but may also be steamed like spinach and other greens.

Soybeans

Soybeans are one of the most nutritious crops you can grow. What makes them especially valuable is that they are rich in just those nutritional areas in which many other vegetables and fruits are weak, thus forming a good complement to other crops in your garden. They are, for instance, as rich or richer in protein than any other garden crop; only ½ cup of cooked beans provides nearly 10 grams of very high-quality protein. In addition, soybeans are a very rich source of phosphorus, iron, potassium, and thiamine and a good source of calcium. They are also rich in lecithin,

Superior Sweet Potato Varieties

Sweet potatoes are considered to be an outstanding source of vitamin A, but how much of this vitamin you actually harvest depends on the variety you plant. Centennial, the most popular sweet potato variety grown in North America, is also one of the very richest in vitamin A. Ratings published in 1965 showed both Centennial and Julian as containing 18 milligrams of carotene per 100 grams. Following these top two varieties were Goldrush (12 milligrams per 100 grams), Heart O'Gold, Georgia Red, Kandee, and Porto Rico (all with 6 milligrams per 100 grams). Two varieties, White Star and Pelican Processor, failed to show any significant amounts of vitamin A.[4] Not included in this study was the variety Allgold, which shouldn't be overlooked by gardeners. Allgold has roughly three times the vitamin A of the variety Porto Rico. In general, a deeper shade of orange in the flesh of the sweet potato indicates greater carotene content and vitamin A activity.

which has shown an ability to break up cholesterol and other fatty substances in the body.

Soybeans are one of the most versatile of vegetable crops. They can be eaten cooked, like other beans, but also toasted, like peanuts, ground into flour or grits, made into soy milk or soy cheese, or made into a variety of other products to serve as a meat substitute. Because of their delicate flavor, soybeans quickly pick up the flavors of foods they are cooked with and thus can serve as a base for recipes calling for a wide variety of other, stronger-tasting vegetables and herbs. Soy products can turn almost any dish into one that's good tasting and high in protein.

Eat-All Squash

The flesh of Eat-All squash is, like other winter squash, rich in vitamin A, riboflavin, and potassium. Unlike other winter squash, however, Eat-All has a surprise nutritional bonus. The seeds have no hulls, so they can be left in the squash when it is baked and eaten, or they may be removed and roasted like sunflower seeds. These seeds are fully 35 percent protein and rich in minerals. Eat-All (also called Sweet Nut squash) is certainly worth a try in the home garden.

Jersey Golden Acorn Squash

Jersey Golden Acorn, a 1982 All-American selection, is a bush, acorn-type squash with a vitamin A bonus. It contains about three times as much A as the standard green acorn varieties, putting it up near butternut squash, which is unequaled among squashes for vitamin A content. It may be eaten in the immature state as a summer squash or left to mature into a true winter squash for long-term storage. Its vitamin A content increases with maturity, however, as indicated by the orange flesh, which grows deeper in color (the sign of carotene development) as the season progresses. If you have traditionally grown acorn squash, try Jersey Golden Acorn for a three-fold vitamin A bonus.

Kuta Squash

Kuta is a wonderfully versatile squash that offers up to 100 percent more phosphorus and calcium than other types of squash and good amounts of potassium and vitamins A and C, as well.

Introduced in 1981 by Park Seed Company, this hybrid is compact in form, easy to grow, and a prolific producer. The young fruit can be used as tender summer squash, eaten cooked or raw, shell and all. Or the young, light green fruit can be left to mature on the vine into a true hard-shelled winter squash. In addition, Kuta retains a firm texture when canned or frozen and is a good winter keeper, making it a truly all-purpose—and highly nutritious—addition to the ranks of squash varieties.

Mammoth Russian Sunflower

Sunflowers belong in every garden. Their seeds are certainly among the most nutritious of all garden products, offering highly concentrated amounts of vitamins and minerals in every handful. As a snack or as an addition to many recipes, they can't be beat.

Based upon a ¼-cup serving, sunflower seeds are the third richest garden crop in protein content, by far the richest in phosphorus, second in iron content (trailing only amaranth), third in zinc, first by far in thiamine, and fourth in niacin. In addition, sunflower seeds are the best source of the essential fatty acids (vitamin F) and are especially high in linoleic acid, the most essential of the essential fatty acids. The seeds are about 46 percent fat in the form of a 91.5 percent unsaturated acid, almost a perfect oil for human needs. Sunflower seeds also provide up to 31 units of vitamin E in every 3½ ounces and are a rich source of vitamin D, which is present in very few other foods. It's interesting to note that the protein of the seeds is high in the essential amino acid methionine, which is weak in nearly all other vegetable crops. This trait makes sunflower seeds an especially valuable component of vegetarian meal plans.

Although all sunflowers produce seeds of nearly equal nutritional value, perhaps the most rewarding variety to grow is the Mammoth Russian. This is the tallest of all the sunflower plants, often reaching a height of 12 feet or more, bearing enormous flower heads filled with large, striped seeds that are thin shelled, meaty, and flavorful. Considering that sunflowers are so easy and such fun to grow (not to mention their outstanding nutritional rewards), there's no excuse for not finding room for these vigorous plants. Place them along the northern border of the vegetable garden (where they won't shade other crops) or anywhere there's an unused, sunny spot on the home grounds.

Caro-Red and Caro-Rich Tomatoes

In 1958, scientists at Purdue University developed Caro-Red, an orange-fleshed tomato with about ten times the vitamin A content of standard tomatoes. To get the new A-rich variety, they crossed common tomatoes with the South American "wild hairy" tomato, which was especially vitamin rich. Caro-Red resembles the popular tomato variety Rutgers except that its skin is orange, its flesh orange-red, and its taste somewhat different from—but not inferior to—other garden tomatoes. Because of its low acid content, people who've tasted this variety claim that it is sweeter flavored than standard tomatoes.

In 1974, Purdue released an improved variety, Caro-Rich. While retaining the same high nutritional quality as Caro-Red, the new variety features larger fruits, more crack resistance, and resistance to fusarium wilt, and its taste is more like that of conventional tomatoes.

Doublerich Tomato

New Hampshire plant breeders crossed a tiny, wild, Peruvian tomato, extremely high in vitamin C content, with several common garden tomatoes to achieve the Doublerich, a variety that looks like other tomatoes

---

Superior Watermelon Varieties

While watermelons may not be the best garden source of vitamin A you can grow, they can still be considered an above-average source. The variety of watermelon you select will have some bearing on the amount of vitamin A present. According to a 1963 study, Charleston Gray was the variety richest in vitamin A. It contained 0.60 milligrams of carotene per 100 grams of fruit, compared to 0.54 milligrams for Mandella, 0.14 milligrams for Candy Red, 0.36 milligrams for Strawberry, 0.11 milligrams for Royal Golden, and 0.14 milligrams for Purdue Hawkesbury.[5] In general, a deeper red color in the fruit signifies higher vitamin A content in watermelons.

but contains twice the amount of vitamin C. While ordinary tomatoes have from 15 to 25 milligrams of vitamin C in a 3½-ounce fruit, Doublerich has 50 milligrams, meaning that one medium-size Doublerich tomato alone comes close to satisfying the Adult Recommended Dietary Allowance (60 milligrams).

The ascorbic acid of Doublerich has real staying power when the fruits are canned, frozen, or made into juice. USDA tests show that juice from Doublerich retains nearly all of its vitamin C after one year of storage in sealed canning jars. Doublerich juice, then, is comparable in C content to orange juice. With Doublerich, there is good reason for temperate-climate gardeners to break the orange juice habit and get their breakfast ration of vitamin C directly from the home garden.

CHAPTER 3

Building Soil for Nutrition

Up until the time a tomato is harvested and appears on the dinner table, it receives sustenance from the soil. Nearly all gardeners, somewhere in their hearts, believe that the quality of that tomato on the dinner table has something to do with the quality of the soil in which it was grown. And, indeed, it does. But the relationship between soil character and food quality is a complex one, little understood by agronomists or nutritionists. And what *is* understood about this relationship might sometimes surprise you.

Why is so little actually known about the soil connection? You might gain some insight from the following statement made by a major California lettuce producer.

> *I don't care what's on it, or what's in it, or what it tastes like, so long as it is in the right shape and the right number will pack into a box and the box will pass the inspector.*[1]

For the most part, the commercial grower tends to give little thought to the nutritional quality of the food he raises. He cares more about yield and ease of shipping the product to market, the two factors critical to his profit margin. Agronomists do not concern themselves with nutrition in crops since they work primarily to serve the grower's interests. And nutritionists, although they obviously care about nutrition, have very little to say about soil management practices.

Who does that leave to care? *You.* You are the one who cares about the nutritional quality of the food you eat, and the surest and most direct way to get quality food is to grow it yourself. And when you're gardening for nutrition, that means starting with the soil.

From Soil to Plant

To put a very complex process into very simple terms, nutrient salts from the soil are taken up by a plant's roots and travel in solution up the plant's vascular system to the foliage, where they are combined and converted into plant tissues. However, most of a plant's food—up to 95 percent—is manufactured without the aid of soil elements. In the presence of light, the green parts of the plant draw carbon dioxide from the air and water from the roots, converting these into sugar, which is then used for energy production or is stored, often in the form of starch, for future use. The mineral elements from the soil are needed in relatively small amounts—sometimes infinitesimal amounts—and yet, the lack of any necessary one of them will affect the plant and often will affect the nutritional quality of its food portion.

Some agricultural scientists have made the statement that the quality of a food has little, if anything, to do with the quality of the soil. If any plant does not get what it needs from the soil, they argue, it will simply not grow, and if it does get everything it needs, then the food crop will have all the nutrition it is supposed to have. This is a neat little bit of logic with only one flaw. It's not true.

First of all, the nutrient needs of plants are not the same as those of human beings. A healthy plant, with all its needs fulfilled, does not necessarily offer a good nutritional package for people. Take one small example, iodine. This element is critical in human nutrition as a regulator of the thyroid gland. Without it, we would develop goiter. Yet, except for some seaweeds, plants do not need it. Much of the iodine naturally present in Midwestern soils in the United States was drained away during the last ice age, and as a result of this soil deficiency, many Midwesterners developed goiter. The federal government, making the connection, didn't move to replace iodine in the soil, but instead decided to force salt manufacturers to add iodine to their product, figuring that everyone uses salt. The result is that today goiter is rarely seen, although, ironically, salt-related heart disease has become virtually endemic among the American population.

Another example is fluorine, not essential for plants but known to play a role in human nutrition. After World War II, it became fashionable for local governments to add fluorine to public drinking water to help prevent tooth decay in children. This was added in the form of sodium fluoride, a volatile toxic substance. According to David Reuben, M.D., writing in his book *Everything You Always Wanted to Know about Nutrition* (Simon and Schuster, 1978), the maximum safe dosage of fluorine is 1 milligram a day. Yet, fluoridated water will add 1.6 milligrams to the daily diet. A fluoridated toothpaste will add another milligram, and normal food intake contributes about 0.45 milligrams. All together, these add up to more than three times the maximum safe dosage as established by the U.S. Public Health Service. When a nutritional deficiency is detected, the government tends to ease it not by improving agricultural soils, as might seem the reasonable way, but by broadcasting the substance to the populace at large, in various and wondrous ways.

Some other trace elements—sodium, vanadium, silicon, cobalt, and selenium—are needed by only some plant species but are necessary to complete human nutrition. Fortunately, the government has not yet decided to add these to our drinking water (although you will receive considerable and potentially harmful doses of sodium if your water is artificially softened).

Second, it is not true that a plant will not draw up and store elements that are not needed for its growth. If iodine or fluorine are available in the soil, the plant will draw them up whether it needs them or not. This makes it possible for you to assure that the optimum amounts of trace minerals are present in your food crops (even if these elements are not needed for plant nutrition) by assuring their presence in the soil.

Third, any fruit or vegetable cannot be counted on to have the nutritional quality it is supposed to have, according to United States Department of Agriculture (USDA) food charts. It's not true that the plant will simply refuse to grow if the full nutritional complement is not obtained from the soil. Often, the plant will grow just the same— sometimes not as large and lush, but other times looking just the same as a fully nourished crop. It depends on the particular nutrient and its specific role in the plant.

The content of mineral elements varies tremendously from one soil to another, not only among different sections of the country, but among fields only a few miles from each other, or even side by side. Not surprisingly, these deficiencies or abundances are often reflected in the nutritional quality of the crops grown on those soils. One study in Idaho revealed concentrations of calcium in cattle forage plants ranging from 0.50 to 2.84 percent of the dry matter, depending on the field selected.[2] That's a difference of 568 percent in calcium content! When it came to phosphorus content, the difference was 292 percent. Measuring trace elements, researchers found a 450 percent difference in cobalt, 400 percent in copper, 740 percent in manganese, and 260 percent in zinc.

(Many of the studies relating to plant nutrition, incidentally, are concerned with cattle forage crops. Much less study has been done with human food crops. One reason, of course, is that there is good commercial profit in feeding cattle well and very little in feeding humans well. And since the cattle now seem to be well fed, it seems incumbent upon us to do as well for our own nutritional needs.)

There have been many cases in our nation's history where local populations, particularly children, have developed deformities and other illnesses related to the poor quality of local soils. We have prided ourselves on putting these dark chapters behind us, wiping out rickets and other gross deficiency diseases by generally upgrading the nation's prosperity and by making available foods from various parts of the country, where one soil's deficiencies may easily be compensated for by foods from other regions.

Now, however, we seem to be taking giant steps backward, this time on a national scale. Instead of obtaining all our food from our own small locality, as many families did during the years of the Great Depression, we are depending on foods grown commercially in increasingly concentrated sunbelt areas, where the chances of soil depletion grow greater each year. The general attitude of the agribusiness executives who grow your super-market produce is to treat the soil as an inert substance and to force-feed the chemicals needed to produce salable products. As the California grower said, "I don't care what's on it, or what's in it, or what it tastes like. . . ." Florida citrus growers, working with nutrient-poor, sandy soil, force-feed their trees from crop to crop. They will add those trace elements necessary to produce oranges either by running nutrients through the sand or by spraying them on the foliage, but producing a nutritious crop is not their overriding concern. And, in fact, one study found that Valencia oranges grown in the sandy soils of Florida had only one-third as much vitamin A as Valencias grown in the richer soils of California.[3]

The important lesson for the gardener is this: the more you depend on your own crops for nutritional needs, the more you must be certain that your soil contains optimum amounts of all the nutrients needed for both plant and human needs. You'll find more about supplying these needs later in this chapter.

How Important Is NPK?

Nitrogen, phosphorus, and potassium—otherwise known as NPK—are the big three in plant nutrition. How important are they to producing nutritious crops? The answer is—not as important as you might think.

Commercial fruit and vegetable growers keep their soils well supplied with NPK, often with the addition of calcium. And the crops they raise today are no more nutritious than those our grandparents grew. In fact, of all the many factors that affect the nutritional quality of fruits and vegetables, NPK decidedly takes a back seat. Let's look at some of the other factors that can have an impact on nutritional quality.

Variety: The variety of the crop often makes a major difference in its nutritional makeup. Unfortunately, there has been precious little research done to compare standard varieties of common crops—Nantes versus Danvers carrots, white versus purple eggplants, the more than 50 available strains of cabbage, and so on. The nutritional content of new hybrids is not listed in the seed catalogs either. Nutritional comparisons and nutritional listings aren't likely to become a regular feature in seed-catalog descriptions in the near future. Still, you should continue to scour the catalogs each season, looking for signs of new high-vitamin, high-mineral varieties. Gardening magazines often feature articles on up-and-coming varieties, which can also aid you in your search.

Soil structure: Whether or not a particular soil has a good supply of calcium is of little importance if the soil is basically unable to deliver that calcium to plants. Clearly then, the structure of the soil plays a paramount role in delivering nutrition to plants. A soil rich in organic matter, earthworms, and microorganisms will have good structure. In good garden loam, the individual particles of sand, clay, and silt group together into larger particles called granules or aggregates. The granules create a good crumb structure that promotes aeration and holds water. Soil nutrients are held in soluble form in this water and are pulled into plant tissues through the roots by capillary action. Sandy soils lack the organic matter content to hold the nutrient-laden water where plant roots can get to it. Both

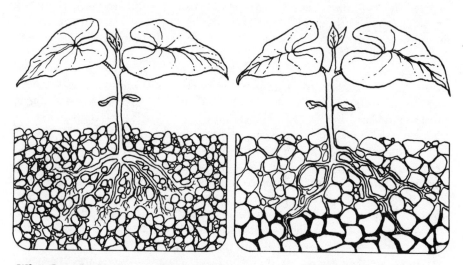

What Goes On Underground: *In the loamy soil on the left, plants will be well nourished, since nutrient-laden moisture is held in the root zone by the good "crumb" structure. In the sandy soil at right, plants will languish, since the poor soil structure allows soluble nutrients to seep down below the reach of the plant roots.*

moisture and the mineral salts are soon carried beyond the root zone by leaching, or up into the atmosphere by evaporation. (This explains why commercial crops grown on sandy soils must be fed constantly through liquid solution or foliar sprays.) In your garden, work first for high organic content and good soil structure, which in turn promote efficient nutrient use by garden crops.

Rainfall and soil moisture: There have been several experiments which measured the effects of rainfall and soil moisture on the vitamin C content of crops. In every experiment the same pattern emerged. The drier the soil, the higher the vitamin C content—15 percent more in potatoes, up to 33 percent more in turnip greens. But the researchers also found that the yield of the crop was reduced in the dry soils. So you can take your choice— smaller potatoes richer in vitamin C or larger potatoes poorer in vitamin C. It seems that the large amount of water taken up by the crops did not bring along with it the soil components for the manufacture of extra ascorbic acid, even though it did prompt high yields.

Temperature: Experiments in this area have shown no conclusive results at all. In certain studies, some food crops produced slightly more vitamin C at higher temperatures, while others produced more at lower temperatures. For now, we must conclude from the little evidence we have that temperature is not a telling factor. This is good news for gardeners who are attempting to add to fall nutritional yields by growing greens in cold frames that hold temperatures just above the minimum needed for plant growth. It also comes as good news to those who are concentrating on outdoor fall plantings of cold-resistant Chinese vegetables. You aren't jeopardizing nutrient value when you expose hardy plants to low temperatures.

Light: Light duration and intensity, more than any other factor, seem to play a direct role in the nutritional quality of crops. Ascorbic acid production is certainly a light-associated process. If a leafy crop is placed in total darkness for 24 hours, it will lose up to 20 percent of its ascorbic acid (a fact to remember when storing crops). Experiments with tomatoes, peas, peppers, turnip greens, and kale all show the same pattern. Crops harvested later in the season, when the days are shorter, have significantly less vitamin C than those harvested in late spring or early summer, when days are longest. This factor becomes more important as latitude increases, so gardeners in the north are affected more by this factor than are those further south, where daylength differences are less.

In the garden, turnip greens which were shaded from direct sun by a canvas canopy for only 4½ days prior to harvest had only 69 percent as much vitamin C as unshaded plants right next to them.[4] Tomatoes that

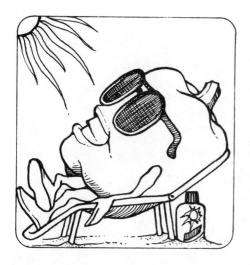

More Sun Means More Vitamin C:
The more sun your crops soak up, the more vitamin C they'll deliver to the dinner table.

were shielded from the sun by the plant's foliage had 37 percent less vitamin C than those tomatoes that ripened in full sun.[5] Beans that were planted too close together likewise suffered vitamin C losses. And the green outer leaves of cabbages are known to have 13 times as much vitamin C as the palest inner leaves.[6]

So far, all the evidence concerns vitamin C. But vitamin A is involved, too. As reported in volume 20 of *Plant Physiology*, turnips grown in late spring and early summer contain significantly more carotene (the precursor to vitamin A) than those grown in late summer and early fall. They also contain twice as much iron. These experiments were carried out in Ithaca, New York, where daylength decreases significantly from June until September.

The lessons to nutrition-conscious gardeners are these: avoid crowding plants in the garden so there's no unnecessary shading; allow sunlight to reach ripening fruits insofar as possible; and try to harvest crops after a few days of full sun. If you harvest after four or five days of cloudy and rainy weather, you won't be gaining optimum nutrition. It's important to realize that vitamin C content will rise again when the sun begins to shine. If you wait for a few sunny days, then make your harvest, the vitamin C content of crops should have regained its previous level.

If you're a northern gardener, you should be happy to hear of these findings. In the higher latitudes, summer days are longer and crops can build up maximum concentrations of vitamin C, carotene, iron, and presumably some other nutrients, as well. You are compensated, at least in part, for your short growing season by the opportunity to raise particularly nutritious crops.

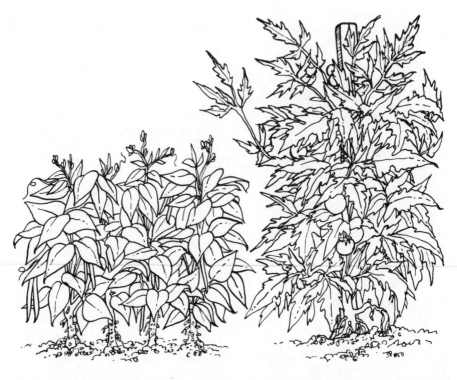

Lessons To Be Learned: *Overcrowding in the bush bean patch, at left, can lower the vitamin C content of your beans. A poorly pruned tomato plant with clusters of fruit shaded by dense foilage will also yield a less than optimum supply of C. To get the most nutrition out of the garden, avoid overcrowding and let ripening crops bask in as much sun as possible.*

The Critical Balance

Nitrogen, phosphorus, and potassium applied to the soil will certainly increase yields, but they do not always enhance the nutritional quality of crops. In fact, the force-feeding of crops with chemical forms of these major nutrients, without regard to the balance of all nutrients, can sometimes actually lower nutritional quality.

One experiment showed that synthetic nitrogen fertilizer, in this case sodium nitrate, increased the protein content of some crops but decreased their mineral content.[7] Writing in an issue of the *Journal of Applied Nutrition*, Dr. Walter Ebeling stated:

> *The addition of the usual "complete" fertilizer (NPK or NPKCa) to depleted soils always increases productivity but does not always increase the nutritive value of the crop. In fact the level of*

certain nutrients may be reduced by dilution caused by the more rapid growth of plant tissue.[8]

Nitrogen fertilizer increased yields of turnip greens but decreased their vitamin C content. In tests with grains, chemical nitrogen decreased the content of some essential amino acids, including lysine, in wheat, barley, rye, and oats. This served to reduce their overall nutritional value.

In an experiment comparing chemically and organically grown potatoes, the chemically grown potatoes showed higher fresh yields.[9] But, during winter storage, the chemically raised tubers had a much greater moisture loss, so eventual *real* yields were higher on the organic side. In this case, chemical fertilization without regard to nutrient balance brought about high moisture content and poorer nutritional quality—both characteristics of *empty* growth.

The fact that overfeeding with nitrogen causes crops to grow large, lush, and nutritionally deficient was demonstrated in an even more striking way by an experiment conducted by German scientists in 1974. They made random selections of the largest red cabbages they could find (weighing up to 5½ pounds) and compared them to the smallest heads that were available (ranging from 5 to 9 ounces). The huge cabbages had only 5 percent of the vitamin C, based on fresh weight, of the small cabbage heads.

Recent experiments at the Rodale Research Center in Maxatawny, Pennsylvania, showed some surprising results when various nitrogen fertilizers were used with green, leafy food crops. Chicken-manure tea was used to fertilize one planting of Chinese celery cabbage while ammonium nitrate, a commonly used and readily available chemical form of nitrogen, was used to fertilize another. When the mature plants were analyzed, the chemically fed group was found to have four times as much nitrate (indicating inefficient use of nitrogen) as the organically fed group, while the organic vegetables had nearly double the vitamin C level of their chemically grown counterparts. These striking results give strong indication that organic forms of nitrogen are more easily handled by growing plants than rapidly acting chemical forms. Other experiments, comparing organic fish-emulsion fertilizer with ammonium nitrate in test plots of chard, lettuce, and spinach, yielded similar results. The lesson here is clear. If you feed your garden crops with slow-release, organic forms of nitrogen instead of chemical compounds, your crops will build up more vitamin C and have lower levels of nitrate, a substance which is suspected of posing health hazards in the human diet.

A disregard for nutritional balance in the soil can have other deleterious effects. All the soil nutrients, both major and minor, work in interrelated ways to provide plant nutrition. To disturb this relationship through thoughtless fertilization practices usually harms both soil and plants. An excess of phosphorus, for example, can lead to an iron or zinc deficiency.

An excess of either iron or manganese can induce a deficiency of the other. Excess nitrogen brings about a deficiency of phosphorus, sulfur, and copper. An overabundance of chlorine can lead to a nitrogen deficiency. Other nutrients having critical effects on each other are, according to Dr. Ebeling, magnesium–phosphorus, potassium–nitrogen, calcium–nitrate, iron–copper, zinc–phosphorus, zinc–selenium, and calcium–boron.

Balance, among both macronutrients and micronutrients, is the key to a fertile soil and nutritious crops. The normal agricultural practice of applying generous amounts of NPK and supplying only those trace elements necessary to maintain yields has led to poorer soils and poorer crops. As Dr. Ebeling says:

> *Experiments conducted with due consideration of the* balance *[his emphasis] of nutrients in the soil have shown that fertilization can have a profound effect on the nutritive value of plant crops . . . . In any case, the agronomist and the farmer are rarely concerned with the nutrient composition of a crop. Varieties, cultural practices, and fertilizers are all decided on the basis of yield expectation.*[10]

The Role of Micronutrients

Of the micronutrients, boron seems to be especially important to plant nutrient content. A positive relationship was found between this element and the carotene content of carrots. A deficiency of boron was associated with a strikingly lower level of both carotene and riboflavin in tomatoes. Other experimenters found that the combination of boron and manganese increased the ascorbic acid content of cabbage, lettuce, and snap beans.

Magnesium is especially important to plant development since it is necessary for photosynthesis. Large amounts are needed in order for plants to produce oils and fats (and the vitamins found in them) and to draw up phosphorus from the soil. Phosphorus, important to human nutrition, is needed in larger quantities by humans than by plants. A high concentration of calcium and potassium, as might be applied by chemical means, depresses the plant's absorption of magnesium. This in turn hinders the plant's ability to take up phosphorus. Again, this is a case where imbalance in soil nutrients affects the nutritional quality of plants.

Sulfur is needed for the synthesis of the amino acids cystine, cysteine, and methionine and for the synthesis of protein itself. Without sufficient supplies of sulfur, plants will not develop good supplies of these amino acids, and the quality of the protein will be greatly lowered. (Keep in mind that the amino acids needed for good plant growth are not the same as those required for good human growth—the plants may flourish but not carry in them the amino acids that humans need.) To improve the quality of all plant proteins, insofar as possible, a steady supply of sulfur is needed in the soil. Gypsum is a rich source of sulfur, although some organic gardeners question its use. Alfalfa readily pulls up sulfur from the soil and stores it in its tissues. You can keep your soil supplied with sulfur by adding alfalfa to the compost or by turning under an alfalfa hay mulch every year. And if there is a silver lining to the cloud of acid rain, it is this—industrial pollutants do contribute sulfur to the soils on which they fall. Gardeners in industrial areas can take at least some solace in this small offering. Last, be aware that microorganisms are necessary to transform sulfur into a form plants can use. A soil rich in decaying organic matter will offer the billions of microorganisms needed for this task.

Selenium, an essential element needed in minute amounts by the human body, has been associated with the prevention of cancer. The two groups of food plants richest in selenium are grains and the brassicas (a group that includes broccoli, Brussels sprouts, cabbage, cauliflower, Chinese cabbage, collards, kale, kohlrabi, mustard greens, and turnips). Among the brassicas, broccoli is the most outstanding source. Soils in certain areas are low in selenium, but any deficiency can be corrected by adding animal manures to the compost.

Zinc is a critical micronutrient, and it is often deficient in soils, even those fertilized heavily with nitrogen, phosphorus, and potassium. In fact, there is evidence that large introductions of NPK can tie up zinc and make it unavailable to plants. This can have serious consequences for plant growth; corn grown in soil lacking zinc shows a lack of tryptophan, one of the essential amino acids. Zinc is also vitally important to the growth process in animals and is associated with protein formation. To be sure your garden has its full share of this important mineral, work lots of organic matter into the soil; organic-rich soils are seldom deficient in zinc.

The overliming of soils (shifting the pH from acid to alkaline) can have unpredictable results. This practice can lead to iron deficiency in the soil, which can be carried right into the crops grown there. In iron-deficient soils in Florida, the iron content of turnip greens was only 22 percent as high as that of turnip greens grown on normal soils. Overliming can also lead to soil (and plant) deficiencies of zinc and manganese.

Organic Soil Building to the Rescue

Nutrient balance is the key to good soils and good crops. And the sure road to nutrient balance is a steady program of organic soil building.

Soil nutrients in organic matter are released as they are needed by plants. There's no chance for a plant to get an unbalanced application of certain nutrients unless the soil itself is deficient in one or more of the nutrients. We have already seen in an earlier section, The Critical Balance, just what chemical nitrogen fertilizers can do to the nutrient balance of the soil and the nutritional quality of crops. Organic matter, on the average, contains about 5 percent nitrogen, which is released slowly as the organic matter decays under the action of microorganisms. The same process takes place with all soil nutrients available in organic matter as well as in natural rock powders, such as phosphate rock and granite dust, which are often added to soils or compost for their special mineral properties.

Because of the natural way they are delivered to plants, you can think of the nutrients in organic matter as being prebalanced. The plant is not forced to accept nutrients it would not, under natural conditions, take from the soil. This nearly perfect balance translates into foods of superior nutritional quality, as demonstrated by many experiments.

F. A. Gilbert, in his book *Mineral Nutrition and the Balance of Life* (University of Oklahoma Press, 1957), reported that turnip greens grown in soils high in organic matter averaged more than 250 percent of the iron found in greens grown in soils low in organic matter.

Dr. Dietrich Knorr, a nutritionist at the University of Delaware, reported on his findings comparing organically grown foods (which he termed eco-foods) to those grown by conventional (meaning chemical) methods. Using laboratory animals as subjects, he found that millet and wheat grown with manure were of a significantly higher nutritional quality than those grains grown with conventional chemical fertilizers. Here's a look at other findings reported by Dr. Knorr:

> A three year study with rabbits compared the effect of a "common diet" which was a commercial preparation with one of similar components that were ecologically grown (wheat, carrots, oats, hay). The number of animals born alive was significantly higher and also the number of animals alive after 90 days was highest when fed with the "organic" diets. The percentage of animals born dead was highest in the "common" diet group.[11]

> The results of Schuphan's 12-year experiment gave a dry matter content for the eco-foods which was 23% higher than the one for conventionally grown foods.[12]

> Some of the essential amino acids of barley protein decreased when nitrogen fertilizer application was increased from 0 to twice the optimum amount. McCarrison as well as Pettersson showed that the protein content was lower after NPK application when compared to "organic" fertilizer application.[13]

> Higher vitamin C concentrations for eco-foods were recorded as a result of long term experiments by Schuphan, and about 3.6 times more vitamin C and 2.3 times more B-carotene were found in ecologically grown leeks and carrots respectively. Ecological farming increased the iron uptake of spinach significantly over mineral fertilizer application.[14]

In other experiments, organically grown kale had 93 percent more ascorbic acid than its chemically grown counterpart. The vitamin C content of spinach was increased by 89 percent, cabbage by 13 percent, Brussels sprouts by 47 percent, kohlrabi by 13 percent, and endive by 36 percent when grown organically instead of chemically.[15]

Arrowhead Mills, in Deaf Smith County, Texas, has been growing organic wheat for many years. Now, working with a soil long converted to organic methods, they have compared independent analyses of their own wheat to average wheat as expressed in the standard USDA food tables. The results say it all: the organically grown wheat was found to be up to 69 percent richer in protein.[16]

Getting Started

The first step to improved garden soil is a complete soil test. Home testing kits, available commercially, are useful for gauging rough levels of nitrogen, phosphorus, potassium, and pH, but a test conducted by your state soils laboratory will be more accurate and will include assays (analyses) of the micronutrients, as well. The test will cost a few dollars, but it will be an investment well made, especially if you plan to depend on your garden for a greater proportion of your nutritional needs. For details on how to collect and submit a soil sample, call or write your local agricultural or horticultural agent.

If the test shows a major deficiency of any element, then you should take immediate steps to supply that element to your soil, using an organic

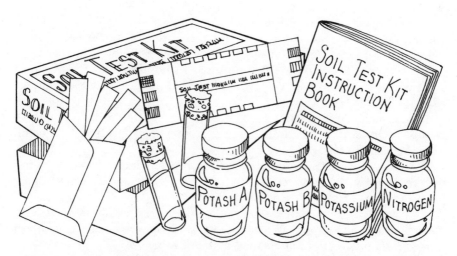

Do-It-Yourself Testing: *For a quick, rough estimate of the NPK levels in your garden soil and a check on the pH level, a home soil test kit comes in handy.*

material or natural rock powder that's a good source. If your soil has at least acceptable levels of all the macronutrients and micronutrients, then you should simply undertake a general soil-building program that will gradually raise the levels of all nutrients. The chart at the end of the chapter, Soil Health Guide, lists the organic materials that are prime sources of the macronutrients and micronutrients. It also lists nutrient deficiency symptoms that show up in plants, to help you read the health of your soil better.

Composting Materials

Directions for composting are freely given in many other books, and there's no need to go into the composting process in any great detail here. Instead, the emphasis will be on identifying those materials that, working in concert, will provide compost of complete nutritional quality. If, in the past, you have made compost casually, using whatever materials were conveniently available to you, then you will see the job in a different light from now on. You will continue to use all the easily available materials, of course, but you will probably choose to supplement these with other materials that provide specific elements for the nutrition of soil and plants. If you've never before selected composting materials with the express goal of supplying manganese, selenium, or zinc, you might find yourself doing so in the future—especially if the results of your soil test warrant the special attention. To help you with your selection, turn to the chart at the end of the chapter to see which organic materials supply key nutrients. As a further aid, here's a brief rundown of common compost ingredients and the nutrient contributions they make.

• You probably use manure in your compost now. If you don't, then you should begin immediately since manure is one of the best all-around sources of minerals. The reason is that the nutritional needs of farm animals are not much different from those of humans, and the minerals excreted by these animals can, and should, be recycled in the compost heap.

• Leaves are a common compost ingredient, especially valuable because the roots of trees bring up minerals from deep within the earth and store them in the foliage.

• Grass clippings are ubiquitous in compost heaps. It's a good thing they're so easy to come by, since they're a rich source of nitrogen, potassium, and copper.

• Bone meal is rich in nitrogen and calcium and very rich in phosphorus. A few sprinklings on various layers as you build the compost heap will do much to enrich its total nutrient value.

• Save all your wood ashes, for they are one of the best sources of potassium and calcium.

• If a phosphorus deficiency is a problem in your soil, keep a sack of phosphate rock on hand and add a sprinkling over each layer of compost as the heap builds up.

• Dolomitic limestone (dolomite) is another material that's strongly recommended, for it will add the relatively large amounts of magnesium needed for both crop and human nutrition. Soils in the northeastern United States are often deficient in magnesium.

• Sulfur is rarely deficient in soils. If a soil test reveals a lack, however, you can add adequate amounts indirectly by layering alfalfa hay in the compost pile or more directly by turning under a cover crop of alfalfa hay in the garden. This hay, which contains large amounts of sulfur, will overcome any deficiency problems in your soil. Gypsum is an exceptionally rich source of sulfur, although many organic gardeners question its use.

These key ingredients, from manure to alfalfa hay, will combine to form a nutritionally complete compost, one that will offer your food crops all the materials they need to recombine elements into foods of the highest nutritional quality.

In addition to composting, of course, you should continue with other good soil-building practices, including green manuring and the addition of organic materials to build good soil structure. Remember, though, that natural and organic fertilizers are not quick fixes for the soil. They are slow-acting soil builders for the long-term health of the soil. If your test results indicate a severe deficiency of any one element, it may take a full season or more to get your soil back up to a good nutrient level by adding organic materials. But in the end, you will have your own soil bank of nutrients that will contribute, to the greatest extent possible, to healthful foods on your dinner table.

Soil Health Guide

Nutrient	Deficiency Symptoms of Plants	Natural Sources
Nitrogen	Slow growth, slender fibrous stems; pale green or yellow-green color of foliage and stems	Bone meal, dried blood, green manure legume crops
Phosphorus	Reduced vigor, slow growth; red-purple color on undersides of leaves; slow setting of fruit, premature dropping of fruit	Bone meal, manure, phosphate rock
Potassium	Reduced vigor; poor growth; leaves ashen, curled, and bronzed; poorly developed root systems	Basalt rock, granite dust, green plant matter, greensand, manure, wood ashes
Boron	Slow growth; death of terminal buds, then lateral buds; leaves thickened, fruits cracked and discolored; deficiency rare	Apply household borax solution: mix 4 to 5 oz. of borax in 5 gal. of water for 1,000 sq. ft. of soil
Calcium	Retarded growth; development of thick, woody stems; deformities of terminal leaves and young branches	Bone meal, dolomitic limestone, ground oyster shells, limestone, wood ashes
Copper	Slow growth, dieback of shoot tips; deficiency usually on peat or muck soils	Grass clippings, sawdust, wood shavings
Iron	Colorless spots on young leaves; yellow leaves on upper parts of plants; poor growth of new shoots	Greensand, manure
Magnesium	Late and sporadic maturing of plants, yellowing between veins of older leaves, poor fruit quality	Dolomitic limestone; shore dwellers, add 1 qt. of sea water to each 100 lb. of compost

Nutrient	Deficiency Symptoms of Plants	Natural Sources
Manganese	Slow growth, sporadic maturing of plants; areas between veins of leaves turning yellow, then brown, while veins remain green; deficiency likely to occur in highly alkaline soil	Acidic organic matter such as cottonseed meal, oak leaves, oak sawdust, peat moss to lower pH
Selenium	Soil deficiency rare	Manure
Sulfur	Yellowing of leaves (distinguished from nitrogen deficiency because leaves not completely dried out)	Alfalfa hay
Zinc	Leaves abnormally long and narrow, sometimes turning yellow and spotting; often appear together with iron deficiency	Manure, phosphate rock

CHAPTER 4

How Well Can
Your Garden Feed You?

How many of your nutritional needs can you expect the garden to satisfy? Or, to put it another way, just how well can your garden feed you?

The answer depends on several factors which will differ from person to person. How much do you depend on fruits, vegetables, and nuts to serve your present dietary needs? How important a part do other foods—primarily meats, eggs, dairy products, and grains—play in your diet? And what changes, if any, would you like to make in your total diet?

Certainly, it is possible, at least in theory, to get your total nutritional needs, including protein, from the food you grow in your own garden. Almost as certainly, this will not be your goal. Even the self-sufficient homesteader will call upon some foods brought in from the outside to supplement the garden's bounty and probably will take some food supplements for nutritional insurance. But the realization that total self-sufficiency is not only possible, but practicable, will serve to open up a full range of options. What you must do, then, is to fit in your gardening plan with your total lifestyle.

Fruits and Vegetables
in the American Diet

Fruits and vegetables do, of course, play an important nutritional role in our diets. But based upon national consumption patterns, their potential is severely underutilized.

As a nation, we get about half of our vitamin A supply from fruits and vegetables, the rest from meat, poultry, fish, eggs, dairy products, fats, and oils. A 50-year trend shows a sharp decline in consumption of the A-rich fresh vegetables and fruits, a sharp increase in processed forms, and an overall decline in total vitamin A consumption. Certainly, with the wide array of vegetables rich in this vitamin, even the household with a medium-size garden can raise enough produce to supply total vitamin A needs year-round.

Fruits and vegetables supply about 20 percent of our thiamine and niacin, the rest coming primarily from meat, poultry, and fish and also from grains, eggs, and dairy products. However, many of the B vitamins are available in surprisingly rich amounts in a variety of common vegetable crops, so vegetarians need not search out obscure sources, and even the family that wishes merely to cut down on meat will have little trouble filling in with garden sources of the B complex.

We get nearly all of our vitamin C from fruits and vegetables because no other foods contain appreciable amounts of ascorbic acid. However, the long-term trend has been away from fresh fruits and vegetables and toward processed foods, particularly frozen citrus juices. The consumption of fresh potatoes, which used to be an important source of vitamin C as well as many other nutrients, has declined steadily over the past 50 years. But this trend can be reversed, starting in the backyard garden. Through careful planning, gardeners in all climates can raise ample supplies of vitamin C while cutting sharply—or even eliminating—their dependence on supermarket products.

Among other nutrients, we get about one-sixth of our magnesium and one-tenth of our iron from fresh fruits and vegetables. This is an area where the garden can make a significant contribution, for garden products are capable of supplying most of our magnesium and iron needs.

Protein supply is usually a major concern among people who consider cutting down on meat. It's reassuring to know that you can get ample protein by supplementing garden products with whole grains or dairy products.

Vegetables—Capable of So Much More

National consumption patterns show that those fruits and vegetables offering the greatest stores of nutritional goodness are often the ones used least often by consumers. Although we don't want to get into an esoteric discussion of American consumption patterns, a quick survey is important, just to enable you to see how your own household patterns compare with national averages.

When ranked for its total nutritional value among 39 common vegetables and fruits, broccoli comes out on top, according to a survey by two California scientists.[1] But broccoli is used so little that, when ranked for its total nutritional contribution to the American diet, it ranks only twenty-first among the 39 vegetables and fruits considered. Tomatoes ranked number one in total contribution; even though they contain far less total nutrition than broccoli, they are produced and eaten in much greater amounts. Among the other nutrition-rich vegetables that are grossly underutilized are spinach (ranking second in nutritional quality, eighteenth in total nutritional contribution); Brussels sprouts (third in quality and thirty-fourth in contribution); lima beans (fourth in quality and twenty-third in contribution); and peas (fifth in quality and fifteenth in contribution).

Among vitamin A producers, carrots ranked first in both categories. They have plenty of vitamin A, and people eat plenty of them. The other A-rich vegetables that ranked high in the consumption tables are: sweet potatoes (second in quality and second in contribution); spinach (third in quality and seventh in contribution); cantaloupe (fourth in quality and fourth in contribution); and apricots (fifth in quality and eleventh in contribution).

In the vitamin C category, peppers ranked first in nutritional quality but only seventh in total contribution to the American diet. Other vegetables ranking high in vitamin C content were not so popular: broccoli (second in quality and eleventh in contribution); Brussels sprouts (third in quality and twenty-eighth in contribution); cauliflower (fourth in quality and twenty-first in contribution); strawberries (fifth in quality and fourteenth in contribution); and spinach (sixth in quality and twentieth in contribution). Oranges, the seventh most efficient producer of vitamin C, ranked first in total contribution because of the enormous tonnage produced each year.

Among other vitamins, peas ranked highest in niacin, but potatoes made the greatest contribution. Broccoli, spinach, and asparagus were the best sources of riboflavin, but potatoes again contributed the most in total to the diet. Peas, lima beans, and asparagus were individually the most valuable thiamine sources, but potatoes, once again, contributed the most thiamine in total. Lima beans, watermelon, and spinach were the richest in potassium, but—what else?—potatoes contributed the most in total. The same situation occurs with phosphorus, where potatoes were the most important source, even though of lower quality than nine other vegetables including lima beans, peas, and sweet corn, the top-quality sources.

In calcium, potatoes were woefully weak, ranking only thirty-eighth out of 39 fruits and vegetables in calcium content—and yet they ranked first in contribution, again because of the sheer quantity of production and consumption. Broccoli, spinach, and snap beans were ranked first, second, and third in quality but no higher than seventh in total contribution.

The last category is iron, where spinach, lima beans, and peas were the richest sources. Potatoes ranked only nineteenth in quality, but guess which vegetable ranked first in total contribution to the American diet. You should need only one guess by now.

Once all these figures sink in, there are two lessons to be learned. The first is that we are not using many of our most nutritious vegetables as we should. And the second is that we should never underestimate the lowly potato. It is actually an aristocrat in burlap, offering modest amounts of a wide spectrum of nutrients. And we do eat potatoes more often, and in greater amounts at a single sitting, than any other vegetable. The lowly spud is versatile, easy to prepare, and we never seem to grow tired of it. Of course, the potatoes grown in your own garden will be the best, both nutritionally and in taste.

(Before we leave the subject of the California study, here are a few general comments. This study focused on the most commonly consumed foods and thus omitted some that are known to be good sources of particular nutrients. Also, the nutrition calculations the researchers used were based on fresh vegetables. Since more than half of the total potato harvest is converted into potato chips and other convenience foods, at a tremendous loss of nutritional quality, the actual contribution of potatoes may be not quite so important as surmised. Still, we can learn a great deal from the study.)

The Vegetarian Alternative

You may be wondering whether you can get complete protein from the garden, in sufficient amounts. You can if you pay some attention to balancing amino acids. Amino acids, of course, are the building blocks of protein. If any food is low in any one of the essential amino acids, that protein can be used by the human body only to the extent that the supply of the weakest, or limiting, amino acid will allow.

The major garden producers of protein are legumes, sunflowers, and nuts, although broccoli, amaranth, and potatoes offer appreciable amounts. None of these foods by itself offers complete protein, and so vegans (those who choose to eat no foods of animal origin) can combine them with whole grains and soy products, which will fill in the limiting amino acids. And it is even possible to get complete protein in ample amounts by balancing amino acids from garden sources alone, assuming that you can raise whole

(continued on page 52)

What Vitamins and Minerals Do for You

While you are tending your Vitamin A Alley, containing carrots inter-planted with sweet potatoes, or planting your Protein Patch, you might be inspired to consider the ways in which these crops will help you after they disappear from the dinner table. Here is a very brief look at each of the major nutritional elements and the services each performs in the human body.

Protein

This is the basic building substance of the body, critically important to the growth and development of all body tissues. You need it, in good amounts, to replace the worn-out cells of muscles, skin, blood, hair and nails, and all the internal organs. Protein is also needed to form hormones and enzymes, which control all body processes.

Protein is made up of some 20 amino acids, all but eight of which can be produced by the human body. These eight, the essential amino acids, must be obtained from the food you eat. Since all food proteins are broken down in the body into their separate amino acids, then recombined into chains that can be used for human nutrition, it does not matter whether you obtain your protein from animal or vegetable sources. It is the amino acids that are important, not the protein source itself.

Proteins from animal sources are generally of a higher quality (that is, they contain more of the essential amino acids) than those coming from vegetables. But, since many people are attempting to reduce their meat consumption, it is important to realize that complete proteins can be formed by mixing together certain vegetables. This concept is explored further in this chapter under The Vegetarian Alternative.

Vitamin A

This is a fat-soluble vitamin, meaning that it dissolves in fat and can be stored in the fatty tissues of the body. Although you do not need a fresh dietary supply every day, it does take some time to rebuild your vitamin A supply after it has been on the low side for some time.

All of the vitamin A in fruits and vegetables is in the form of provitamin A, or carotene, a substance which is converted into true vitamin A in the human body. Preformed vitamin A is found only in animal sources. This is not to say that preformed vitamin A is preferable to carotene. Indeed, recent medical research indicates that carotene is able to perform some valuable services that preformed vitamin A cannot.

You need vitamin A for healthy skin and for fighting colds and infections. A lack of it can lead to night blindness, sensitivity to glare, difficulty in reading in dim light, and an inability to store fat. People recovering from serious illness or infection need plenty of vitamin A, as does anyone who suffers from a stomach, liver, or intestinal disorder. Children need vitamin A for good growth and dental health.

Vitamin B

This single term actually applies to a fairly large group of different vitamins, some of which have not yet been identified by scientists. Together, they are called the vitamin B complex. Many people do not get enough of some of the B vitamins because they depend on refined white bread and other wheat products which are nutritionally lacking. The majority of the bread and cereal products on the supermarket shelves are first stripped of the bran and germ which contain most of the B vitamins. They are then "enriched" with only three of the B vitamins: thiamine (B_1), riboflavin (B_2), and niacin (B_3).

You need the B complex (all of it) for the health of your digestive tract, skin, mouth and tongue, eyes, nerves, arteries, and liver. The B vitamins are water soluble and cannot be stored in the body for long periods of time. They are destroyed by both light and heat and are easily leached out of foods in the cooking water.

The charts that appear in the section Stars of the Garden, later in the chapter, list ten good garden sources each of thiamine, riboflavin, and niacin. Overall, legumes tend to be the richest sources. Other important members of the B complex are B_6, B_{12}, and folic acid. Peanuts, sunflower seeds, and tomatoes are good sources of B_6 you can raise in the garden. You can supplement these with brewer's yeast, wheat germ, and whole-grain products to make sure your intake of B_6 is adequate. (The Adult Recommended Dietary Allowance [R.D.A.] of B_6 is 2.2 milligrams.) Unfortunately, you can't look to the garden for supplies of B_{12}; this nutrient is found solely in animal sources. Good nongarden sources of B_{12} include eggs, fish, meat, milk, and some fermented soy products such as tempeh. (The R.D.A. for B_{12} is 3.0 milligrams.) Folic acid is in plentiful supply in the garden: asparagus; broccoli; dark green, leafy vegetables (especially collards, spinach, and beet greens); legumes; nuts; and onions provide good amounts. Brewer's yeast is also a good supplementary source of folic acid. (The R.D.A. for folic acid is 400 micrograms.)

Vitamin C

This water-soluble vitamin, also known as ascorbic acid, is a hard one to hold onto. It is easily lost in food processing and cooking, it cannot be stored in the body, and it is easily excreted. In addition, smoking, stress, and exposure to pollutants all destroy vitamin C in the body. It's clear to see that you need to make sure you have a continuing supply to safeguard the health of all body tissues including teeth, gums, bones, blood vessels, and eyes. Above and beyond that, vitamin C protects against infections and colds and is important in recuperation from injury, illness, and surgery.

Fresh garden fruits and vegetables are the best sources of this vitamin. Some of the very best are broccoli, amaranth, and sweet peppers, all of which contain more C than is found in citrus fruits.

Vitamin D

Your body needs this fat-soluble nutrient in order to use calcium and phosphorus efficiently. Although you can't get vitamin D from plant sources, it is plentiful in milk and egg yolks, and your body is capable of manufacturing its own vitamin D from the rays of the sun. Vegans (vegetarians who avoid all foods of animal origin, including milk and eggs) are wise to take a supplemental source of vitamin D.

Vitamin E

This is still a controversial vitamin among scientists. One basic fact is that it's fat soluble, like vitamin A. The general school of thought is that vitamin E is important to heart health and that it acts as an antioxidant,

(continued)

What Vitamins and Minerals Do for You —*continued*

protecting the body's source of vitamins A and C and the unsaturated fatty acids.

Good amounts of vitamin E are found in very few fruits and vegetables, the exceptions being spinach and asparagus. Broccoli leaves contain good amounts, but the flower head that is the desired portion of the plant does not. (The leaves, incidentally, are good to eat and may be added to soups and stews.)

Vitamin E is very easily lost in food processing and in cooking. A study reported in the *American Journal of Clinical Nutrition* (July, 1965) reported that frozen peas contain only 45 percent as much vitamin E as do fresh peas and that canned peas contain only 4 percent as much. Because of the delicate nature of this nutrient and the uncertainty of its supply in foods, many people choose to take a vitamin E supplement.

Iron

As most people know, this nutrient is critical to the health of red blood cells. A lack of it will, indeed, lead to "tired blood." And women need about 80 percent more of it than men.

It's possible to get all your iron from the garden if you plan your meals carefully. The best garden sources are amaranth, dried beans, and other legumes, including lima beans and peas. A more dependable supply comes from occasional servings of beef liver, other beef parts, or a nutritional supplement.

Calcium

The most abundant mineral in the body, calcium plays a paramount role in every life process in both animals and plants. An adult body contains about 3 pounds of calcium, 99 percent of which is deposited in the bones and teeth. The proper functioning of the heart, muscles, nerves, and blood depends on sufficient calcium supplies.

From the garden, you can harvest good supplies of calcium in amaranth, broccoli, collards, kale, and other dark, leafy greens.

Phosphorus

This nutrient forms an important physical component of every living cell. It is necessary for the metabolism of carbohydrates, protein, and fats and critical to the health of blood, teeth, and bones. Milk and cod are excellent

grains and soybeans in your garden. Vegetarians who allow milk, eggs, and cheese into their diets will have no trouble at all in getting adequate amounts of protein, since these foods will provide all the amino acids lacking in garden products.

A food lacking in one or two amino acids can be utilized more fully as protein when it is eaten with a second food which supplies the limiting amino acid. Macaroni and cheese is a good dish because the weak amino sources of phosphorus. Among garden products, the best sources are sunflower seeds, nuts, and legumes.

Potassium

Nerve and skeletal and cardiac muscle function depend on potassium. This nutrient is also essential to children's growth. Deficiencies are uncommon, since ample supplies are available in a wide variety of foods. Chief sources from the garden are potatoes, squash, amaranth, and legumes.

Trace Minerals

Sometimes called micronutrients, these are needed in far smaller amounts than are the macronutrients, but their functions are just as important. A bit of copper is needed for the utilization of iron. Iodine is critical to the thyroid gland for the manufacture of the hormone thyroxine. Manganese must be present to help thiamine do its job. Zinc is necessary for all metabolic functions. Selenium is important to the proper functioning of many enzyme systems. A deficiency of cobalt can lead to anemia. Sodium is essential—but the problem today is how to avoid an excess of sodium, which is loaded into nearly all processed foods in alarming amounts.

You can assure yourself of an adequate supply of all these trace minerals by treating your garden soil with high-quality compost made from a variety of materials. Some soils are naturally deficient in one or more trace minerals, and previously rich soils can become deficient when they are fed nothing but fertilizers containing only the major nutrients nitrogen, phosphorus, and potassium. And if these trace minerals aren't present in the soil, they certainly won't be present in the foods grown in that soil, as chapter 3 clearly points out.

Fiber

You might not think of fiber as a nutritional element, yet it holds an important place in human nutrition. It is a part of foods that is not digested, such as the skin of an apple, the husk of a bean, and the connecting tissues of green, leafy vegetables. Potatoes and sweet potatoes are very rich in fiber. Most refined foods are low in it, particularly refined flour products that have been deprived of the husks (bran) of the wheat kernels. It's worth your while to make sure you get plenty of fiber in your diet. Recent research has linked a low-fiber diet to cancer of the colon and rectum, heart disease, varicose veins, phlebitis, and several other conditions. And because the fiber is not digested, it keeps you feeling fuller on less food, an important element in weight control.

acid in macaroni is strong in cheese, enabling the body to use most of the protein of the macaroni as well as the cheese. If the macaroni were eaten with butter, that protein would be largely lost.

Other good combinations for vegetarians are grains and legumes, seeds and legumes, and milk or eggs with nearly any plant protein. A peanut butter sandwich, on whole-grain bread, with a glass of low-fat milk, is a very good protein combination for adults as well as children.

The essential amino acids are isoleucine, leucine, lysine, methionine, phenylalanine, threonine, tryptophan, valine, and possibly histidine (which, in any case, is essential for children's growth). From *The Vegetarian Alternative*, by Vic Sussman (see Recommended Reading later in this book), we will borrow a list of food groups showing the amino acid strengths and weaknesses of each.

Legumes (beans, peas, lentils)
    Weak: tryptophan, methionine
    Strong: lysine (especially), isoleucine

Grains (wheat, oats, rice, barley, millet, corn, etc.)
    Weak: lysine, isoleucine
    Strong: tryptophan, methionine

Seeds and Nuts (pumpkin, sunflower, sesame, peanut, etc.)
    Weak: lysine, isoleucine (except cashews and pumpkin seeds)
    Strong: tryptophan, methionine

Milk Products
    Weak: none
    Strong: lysine

Eggs
    Weak: none
    Strong: tryptophan, lysine, methionine

Vegetables
    Weak: isoleucine, methionine
    Strong: tryptophan, lysine

Using this list, we can make some interesting comparisons and come up with some good ideas for food combinations. We see that beans are weak in tryptophan and methionine, while grains are strong in these same amino acids. Beans and rice, then, would be a good protein dish. In fact, this combination is a popular one in many parts of the world where meat, milk, and even eggs are scarce.

Vegetables are generally weak in isoleucine and methionine, but beans are strong in these two amino acids. Serve a bean dish with any vegetable, and you will get better protein use from the vegetable.

Other good combinations are whole-grain bread and cheese, wheat bread enriched with soy flour, pea or bean soup served with whole-grain bread, and a legume soup fortified with sunflower meal. If you want to learn more about the amino acid combinations of vegetables and how they can be combined to form complete proteins, read *Diet for a Small Planet* by Frances Moore Lappé (see Recommended Reading later in this book), which goes into the matter in full and interesting detail.

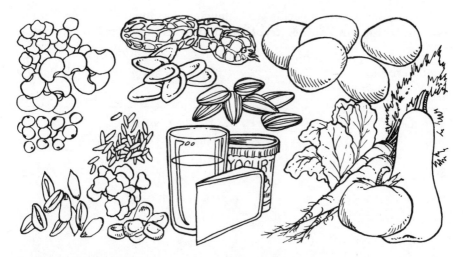

Complementary Proteins: *Each food group has its own amino acid strengths and weaknesses. By learning to balance the amino acids in vegetable and dairy sources, you can come up with combinations that supply complete protein.*

Stars of the Garden

What are the most nutritious crops you can grow in your garden?

You probably know some of them already. Broccoli is widely recognized as a nutritional giant, as are soybeans and sunflower seeds. But some others might surprise you. Lima beans are among the most nutritious vegetables you can grow. Cowpeas and collards, more regional than country-wide favorites, are nutritional powerhouses. Amaranth, a newcomer to North American gardens, is unsurpassed in several nutritional areas. Navy, kidney, and other dry beans shine in many areas. And the potato, as it was pointed out earlier in this chapter, ranks among the most all-around nutritious and versatile of all garden vegetables.

Using United States Department of Agriculture (USDA) data from Agriculture Handbook No. 456, it's possible to rate all the common (and some uncommon) garden crops in 12 nutritional categories: protein, calcium, phosphorus, iron, potassium, vitamin A, thiamine (vitamin B_1), riboflavin (vitamin B_2), niacin (vitamin B_3), vitamin C, magnesium, and zinc. From these results, the top ten crops in each nutritional category can be determined. These winners in each of 12 categories are featured in chart form in the sections that follow. (Because the emphasis of this book is on gardening, not on nutrition alone, these charts will cover only the *major* B vitamins—thiamine, niacin, and riboflavin—and will not go into vitamin B_6 and folic acid.)

Good Protein Sources in the Garden

This listing may surprise you. Have you ever thought of lima beans as a good protein source? They are, as you can see, ranking just a shade behind dry beans in this category.

Ten Good Sources of Protein (*R.D.A. = 45–56 g*)

Crop	Serving Portion	Grams
Soybeans	½ cup, cooked	9.9
Peanuts	¼ cup, roasted, shelled	9.4
Sunflower seeds	¼ cup, raw, hulled	8.7
Lentils	½ cup, cooked	7.8
Navy beans	½ cup, cooked	7.4
Kidney beans	½ cup, cooked	7.2
Great northern beans	½ cup, cooked	7.0
Cowpeas	½ cup, cooked	6.7
Lima beans	½ cup, cooked	6.5
Almonds	¼ cup, raw, shelled	6.1

Other good garden sources: Amaranth, broccoli, peas, potatoes, walnuts

Nongarden sources: Dairy products, eggs, fish, meats, poultry

Good Vitamin A Sources in the Garden

Everybody knows that carrots provide heavy loads of vitamin A. But did you know that a ½-cup serving of baked, mashed sweet potatoes provides more vitamin A than a single 3-ounce carrot? It's true. The other stars of the vitamin A category are winter squash, cress, chard, collards, and, ranking far above the crowd, a crop that you probably don't even plant in your garden—dandelion greens, a bonus gift from your lawn.

Ten Good Sources of Vitamin A (*provitamin A: R.D.A. = 5,000 I.U.*)

Crop	Serving Portion	International Units
Dandelion greens	½ cup, cooked	12,290
Sweet potatoes	½ cup, baked, mashed	9,230
Carrots	1 med., 2⅞ oz., raw	7,930
Collards	½ cup, cooked	7,410
Spinach	½ cup, cooked	7,290
Amaranth	4 oz., raw	6,918
Butternut squash	½ cup, baked, mashed	6,560
Hubbard squash	½ cup, baked, mashed	4,920
Chard	½ cup, cooked	4,725
Garden cress	½ cup, cooked	4,725

Other good garden sources: Apricots, beet greens, broccoli, kale, leaf lettuce, romaine lettuce, muskmelons, mustard greens, New Zealand spinach, peaches, turnip greens, watermelons

Nongarden sources: Dairy products, fish oils (preformed vitamin A), liver

NOTE: *Caro-Rich tomatoes, 1 med., 4¾ oz., raw, is estimated to provide 7,733 I.U.; Jersey Golden Acorn squash, ½ cup, baked, mashed, is estimated to provide 4,305 I.U. No USDA figures are available on these crops.*

Good B-Complex Sources in the Garden

Most people think that the vitamins of the B complex go hand in hand. They often do, when used by the human body, but not necessarily in the garden. Different members of the complex are often supplied by different crops, and your plantings should be planned to provide the widest possible B-complex range. Sunflower seeds are the richest garden source of thiamine, but they don't even rank above average in riboflavin supplies. Broccoli is exceptionally high in riboflavin but only good in thiamine and niacin. Potatoes are an exceptionally good source of niacin but are lacking in riboflavin. For continuing supplies of the entire B complex, choose your crops wisely. (The box on What Vitamins and Minerals Do for You, earlier in this chapter, points out both good garden and good nongarden sources of other noteworthy members of the B complex—namely folic acid, B_6, and B_{12}.)

Ten Good Sources of Thiamine (*vitamin B_1: R.D.A. = 1.2 mg*)

Crop	Serving Portion	Milligrams
Sunflower seeds	¼ cup, raw, hulled	0.71
Cowpeas	½ cup, cooked	0.25
Peas	½ cup, cooked	0.23
Pecans	¼ cup, roasted, shelled	0.23
Soybeans	½ cup, cooked	0.19
Onions	2 oz., dry, raw	0.18
Lima beans	½ cup, cooked	0.16
Okra	4 oz., cooked	0.15
Potatoes	1 med., 7⅛ oz., baked	0.15
Navy beans	½ cup, cooked	0.14

Other good garden sources: Asparagus, avocados, kidney beans, great northern beans, broccoli, dandelion greens and other dark green, leafy vegetables, oranges, peanuts, sweet potatoes, watermelons

Nongarden sources: Beef organ meats, ham, brown rice, whole wheat, brewer's yeast

Ten Good Sources of Riboflavin (*vitamin B$_2$: R.D.A. = 1.7 mg*)

Crop	Serving Portion	Milligrams
Almonds	¼ cup, raw, shelled	0.33
Broccoli	5-oz. stalk, cooked	0.28
Mushrooms	2 oz., raw	0.26
Avocados	½ med., raw	0.23
Okra	4 oz., cooked	0.21
Amaranth	4 oz., raw	0.18
Dandelion greens	½ cup, cooked	0.17
Turnip greens	½ cup, cooked	0.17
Collards	½ cup, cooked	0.14
Winter squash	½ cup, baked, mashed	0.14

Other good garden sources: Asparagus, lima beans, beet greens, Brussels sprouts, chard, sweet corn, cowpeas, garden cress, kale, leaf lettuce, romaine, mustard greens, New Zealand spinach, peas, spinach, summer squash, watermelons

Nongarden sources: Beef organ meats, chicken, dairy products, eggs, ham, wheat germ, brewer's yeast

Ten Good Sources of Niacin (*vitamin B$_3$: R.D.A. = 20 mg*)

Crop	Serving Portion	Milligrams
Peanuts	¼ cup, roasted, shelled	6.2
Potatoes	1 med., 7⅛ oz., baked	2.7
Mushrooms	2 oz., raw	2.4
Sunflower seeds	¼ cup, raw, hulled	2.0
Peas	½ cup, cooked	1.9
Avocados	½ med., raw	1.8
Amaranth	4 oz., raw	1.6
Peaches	1 med., 2¾-in. diameter	1.5
Almonds	¼ cup, raw, shelled	1.3
Cowpeas	½ cup, cooked	1.2

Other good garden sources: Asparagus, lima beans, broccoli, collards, sweet corn, globe artichokes, honeydew melons, kale, muskmelons, okra, rutabagas, summer squash, sweet potatoes, tomatoes, watermelons

Nongarden sources: Beef organ meats, halibut, ham, poultry, rabbit, tuna, whole wheat, brewer's yeast

Good Vitamin C Sources in the Garden

Too many people depend on store-bought citrus fruit for vitamin C when this vitamin can be found in their own backyards. Gardeners in citrus-growing areas are fortunate, indeed, for they can grow their own and get the fruit at its freshest. But gardeners in temperate climes are not without their own backyard resources when it comes to growing ascorbic acid. One small stalk of cooked broccoli contains 40 percent more C than a 6-ounce glass of orange juice. A quarter of a muskmelon provides more vitamin C than half a grapefruit. A 2½-ounce pepper has 12 percent more C than a 7¼-ounce orange. And only four Brussels sprouts have more vitamin C than that same orange. Further, broccoli, muskmelons, peppers, and Brussels sprouts all are much more complete nutritional packages than citrus fruits, which offer little more than vitamin C.

Ten Good Sources of Vitamin C (*ascorbic acid: R.D.A. = 60 mg*)

Crop	Serving Portion	Milligrams
Broccoli	5-oz. stalk, cooked	126
Amaranth	4 oz., raw	91
Sweet peppers	2½-oz. fruit, raw	74
Brussels sprouts	½ cup, cooked (4 sprouts)	68
Oranges	1 med., 2⅝-in. diameter	66
Kale	½ cup, cooked	51
Collards	½ cup, cooked	49
Muskmelons	¼ fruit, 5-in. diameter, 8½ oz.	45
Strawberries	½ cup, 2⅝ oz., whole berries	44
Cabbage	1 cup, raw, finely shredded	42
Grapefruit	½ med., 3⁹⁄₁₆-in. diameter	37
Kohlrabi	½ cup, cooked, diced	36

Other good garden sources: Lima beans, cauliflower, gooseberries, honeydew melons, mustard greens, peas, potatoes, rutabagas, spinach, sweet potatoes, turnip greens, turnip roots, watercress, watermelons

NOTE: *Doublerich tomatoes, 1 med., 4¾ oz., is estimated to provide 68 mg. No USDA data is available on this crop.*

Good Iron Sources in the Garden

When you think of iron, no doubt your thoughts race to Popeye and his iron-rich spinach. But spinach, although a respectable iron source, does not even rank in the top ten. The real providers of iron are dry beans and lima beans, amaranth, and—a surprise—watermelon.

Ten Good Sources of Iron (*R.D.A. = 18 mg*)

Crop	Serving Portion	Milligrams
Amaranth	4 oz., raw	4.4
Navy beans	½ cup, cooked	2.6
Sunflower seeds	¼ cup, raw, hulled	2.6
Great northern beans	½ cup, cooked	2.5
Soybeans	½ cup, cooked	2.5
Butterhead lettuce	4 oz., raw	2.3
Kidney beans	½ cup, cooked	2.2
Lima beans	½ cup, cooked	2.2
Lentils	½ cup, cooked	2.1
Watermelons	1-in.-thick, 10-in.-diameter slice	2.1

Other good garden sources: Almonds, chard, cowpeas, dandelion greens, leaf lettuce, romaine lettuce, peas, spinach, black walnuts

Nongarden sources: Beef, chicken, cod, haddock, blackstrap molasses, turkey, brewer's yeast

Good Phosphorus Sources in the Garden

In general, foods rich in protein are also rich in phosphorus. From the garden, that means seeds, nuts, and legumes—which account for the ten top crops on the phosphorus list. But don't discount the phosphorus value of potatoes even though they are farther down on the list. Because most people eat more potatoes than other vegetables, the common spud may be the most important single phosphorus source.

Ten Good Sources of Phosphorus *(R.D.A. = 800 mg)*

Crop	Serving Portion	Milligrams
Sunflower seeds	¼ cup, raw, hulled	304
Almonds	¼ cup, raw, shelled	164
Black walnuts	1 oz., shelled	162
Soybeans	½ cup, cooked	161
Peanuts	¼ cup, roasted, shelled	147
Navy beans	½ cup, cooked	141
Great northern beans	½ cup, cooked	133
Kidney beans	½ cup, cooked	130
Cowpeas	½ cup, cooked	121
Lentils	½ cup, cooked	119

Other good garden sources: Lima beans, broccoli, potatoes, English walnuts

Nongarden sources: Beef, chicken, cod, dairy products, brewer's yeast

Good Potassium Sources in the Garden

Potassium is important in human nutrition, but it must be balanced with sodium. Excessive intake of table salt can destroy this balance and lead to a potassium deficiency. The lesson to be learned here is to cut down on salt, and increase consumption of these potassium-rich foods. There is no potassium shortage in the garden—and there should be none in your diet.

Ten Good Sources of Potassium

(No recommended dietary minimum, but healthy adults need about 2,500 mg daily)

Crop	Serving Portion	Milligrams
Potatoes	1 med., 7⅛ oz., baked	782
Avocados	½ med., raw	680
Butternut squash	½ cup, baked, mashed	624
Acorn squash	½ cup, baked, mashed	492
Soybeans	½ cup, cooked	486
Amaranth	4 oz., raw	466
Watermelons	1-in.-thick, 10-in.-diameter slice	426
New Zealand spinach	½ cup, cooked	417
Navy beans	½ cup, cooked	395
Great northern beans	½ cup, cooked	375

Other good garden sources: Almonds, apricots, kidney beans, lima beans, broccoli, chard, cowpeas, globe artichokes, honeydew melons, Hubbard squash, butterhead lettuce, leaf lettuce, romaine lettuce, muskmelons, oranges, peaches, spinach, sunflower seeds, sweet potatoes, tomatoes

Nongarden sources: Beef liver, chicken, cod, dairy products, flounder, blackstrap molasses, raisins, salmon, sardines

Good Calcium Sources in the Garden

Spinach has always been touted as a good calcium source, but as you can see in the rankings, it is far inferior to collards, broccoli, turnip greens, and okra. And amaranth has nearly four times the calcium of spinach in an average serving portion. Much of the calcium in spinach, furthermore, is unavailable to the human body because of the high proportion of oxalic acid (oxalate) in this vegetable. Oxalic acid acts to bind the calcium so that it can't be used.

Ten Good Sources of Calcium (*R.D.A. = 1,000 mg*)

Crop	Serving Portion	Milligrams
Amaranth	4 oz., raw	303
Collards	½ cup, cooked	168
Dandelion greens	½ cup, cooked	147
Turnip greens	½ cup, cooked	126
Broccoli	5-oz. stalk, cooked	123
Okra	4 oz., cooked	104
Kale	½ cup, cooked	103
Mustard greens	½ cup, cooked	97
Spinach*	½ cup, cooked	84
Almonds	¼ cup, raw, shelled	83

Other good garden sources: Lima beans, beet greens,* Brussels sprouts, chard,* globe artichokes, leaf lettuce, romaine lettuce, oranges, rhubarb, rutabagas, soybeans, watercress

Nongarden sources: Dairy products, blackstrap molasses, salmon, sardines

*The high proportion of oxalate in beet greens, chard, and spinach make these greens a poor source of available calcium. See the following chart.

Calcium/Oxalate Ratios

Crop	Calcium* %	Oxalate* %	Calcium/ Oxalate Ratio
Worst Calcium/Oxalate Ratios			
Beet greens	0.12	0.92	1:8
Spinach (also New Zealand spinach)	0.12	0.89	1:7
Chard	0.13	0.66	1:5
Best Calcium/Oxalate Ratios			
Broccoli	0.21	0.005	42:1
Collards	0.36	0.009	40:1
Mustard greens	0.24	0.008	30:1
Kale	0.31	0.013	24:1
Turnip greens	0.24	0.015	16:1

*Values for calcium and oxalate contents are expressed as percent dry weight.

SOURCE: *Kohman,* Journal of Nutrition, *18:233, 1939.*

Good Magnesium Sources in the Garden

Since magnesium is an essential element of chlorophyll, it is found in all green, leafy vegetables. But for winter supplies, you can depend on seeds, nuts, and legumes, in which it is even more concentrated. In all seasons, obtaining sufficient magnesium from the garden should be no problem at all.

Ten Good Sources of Magnesium (*R.D.A.* = *400 mg*)

Crop	Serving Portion	Milligrams
Soybeans	¼ cup, dried	138
Cowpeas	¼ cup, dried	98
Almonds	¼ cup	96
Lima beans	¼ cup, dried	81
Pecans	¼ cup, halved	77
Kidney beans	¼ cup, dried	75
Peanuts	¼ cup, roasted, chopped	63
Black walnuts	¼ cup, chopped	60
Beet greens	1 cup, raw, chopped	58
Avocados	½ fruit	56

Other good garden sources: Chard, collards, potatoes, spinach

Nongarden sources: Bananas, blackstrap molasses, Brazil nuts, buckwheat flour, cashews, soy flour, wheat germ

SOURCE: The Complete Book of Minerals for Health *by Sharon Faelten and the Editors of* Prevention *Magazine (Rodale Press, 1981).*

Good Zinc Sources in the Garden

Foods rich in protein are nearly always rich in zinc, as well. Regular consumption of the following seeds, nuts, and legumes, combined with good nongarden sources, will keep every member of the family well supplied with zinc throughout the year.

Ten Good Sources of Zinc (*R.D.A. = 15 mg*)

Crop	Serving Portion	Milligrams
Soybeans	½ cup	3.2
Pumpkin seeds	¼ cup	2.6
Sunflower seeds	¼ cup	2.0
Cowpeas	½ cup	1.5
Peanuts	¼ cup, roasted	1.2
Peas	½ cup, dried, cooked	1.1
Chick-peas	½ cup	1.0
Filberts	¼ cup	1.0
Lentils	½ cup	1.0
Lima beans	½ cup, dried, cooked	0.9

Nongarden sources: Brazil nuts, cashews, fish, meat, poultry, brown rice

SOURCE: The Complete Book of Minerals for Health *by Sharon Faelten and the Editors of* Prevention *Magazine (Rodale Press, 1981).*

All-Star Garden Crops

For your convenience, ten of the preceding charts have been con-
densed into one. At a glance, this chart will tell you in which of the major
nutritional areas each of 89 garden crops shines. Based on the rankings
used in the preceding series of charts, four-star crops are the best of the

All-Star Garden Crops

Crop	Protein	Calcium	Phosphorus	Iron
Almonds	★★	★★	★★★★	★
Amaranth	★	★★★★	—	★★★★
Apples	—	—	—	—
Apricots	—	—	—	—
Asparagus	—	—	—	—
Avocados	—	—	—	—
Beans, great northern	★★	—	★★	★★★
Beans, green snap	—	—	—	—
Beans, kidney	★★★	—	★★	★★
Beans, lima	★★	★	★	★★
Beans, navy	★★★	—	★★★	★★★★
Beans, yellow wax	—	—	—	—
Beet greens	—	★	—	—
Beet roots	—	—	—	—
Blackberries	—	—	—	—
Blueberries	—	—	—	—
Broccoli	★	★★★	★	—
Brussels sprouts	—	★	—	—

★★★★　Exceptionally rich source　　★★　Rich source

★★★　Very rich source　　★　Above-average source

best, ranking in the top three in a particular nutritional category. Three-star crops are nearly as good, ranking in the second group of three. And two-star crops fill out the top ten in each category. The one-star crops are those that missed the top ten list but are, nevertheless, well above average and worthy of planting.

Potassium	Vitamin A	Thiamine	Riboflavin	Niacin	Vitamin C	Total Stars
—	—	—	★★★★	★★	—	15
★★★	★★★	—	★★★	★★	★★★★	24
—	—	—	—	—	—	0
★	★	—	—	—	—	2
—	—	★	★	★	—	3
★★★★	—	★	★★★	★★★	—	11
★★	—	★	—	—	—	10
—	—	—	—	—	—	0
★	—	★	—	—	—	9
★	—	★★	—	★	★	11
★★	—	★★	—	—	—	14
—	—	—	—	—	—	0
—	★	★	★	—	—	4
—	—	—	—	—	—	0
—	—	—	—	—	—	0
—	—	—	—	—	—	0
★	★	★	★★★★	★	★★★★	17
—	—	—	★	—	★★★	5

(continued)

All-Star Garden Crops—*continued*

Crop	Protein	Calcium	Phosphorus	Iron
Cabbage	—	—	—	—
Carrots	—	—	—	—
Cauliflower	—	—	—	—
Celery	—	—	—	—
Chard	—	★	—	★
Cherries, sour	—	—	—	—
Cherries, sweet	—	—	—	—
Chinese cabbage	—	—	—	—
Collards	—	★★★★	—	—
Corn, sweet	—	—	—	—
Cowpeas	★★	—	★★	★
Cucumbers	—	—	—	—
Dandelion greens	—	★★★★	—	★
Eggplants	—	—	—	—
Endive	—	—	—	—
Garden cress	—	—	—	—
Globe artichokes	—	★	—	—
Gooseberries	—	—	—	—
Grapefruit	—	—	—	—
Grapes, Concord	—	—	—	—
Honeydew melons	—	—	—	—
Kale	—	★★	—	—
Kohlrabi	—	—	—	—
Lentils	★★★	—	★★	★★
Lettuce, butterhead	—	—	—	★★★
Lettuce, iceberg	—	—	—	—
Lettuce, leaf	—	★	—	★

Potassium	Vitamin A	Thiamine	Riboflavin	Niacin	Vitamin C	Total Stars
—	—	—	—	—	★★	2
—	★★★★	—	—	—	—	4
—	—	—	—	—	★	1
—	—	—	—	—	—	0
—	★★	★	★	—	—	6
—	—	—	—	—	—	0
—	—	—	—	—	—	0
—	—	—	—	—	—	0
—	★★★	★	★★	★	★★★	14
—	—	—	—	★	—	1
★	—	★★★★	★	★★	—	13
—	—	—	—	—	—	0
—	★★★★	★	★★	—	—	12
—	—	—	—	—	—	0
—	—	—	—	—	—	0
—	★★	—	★	—	—	3
★	—	—	—	★	—	3
—	—	—	—	—	★	1
—	—	—	—	—	★★	2
—	—	—	—	—	—	0
★	—	—	—	★	★	3
—	★	—	★	★	★★★	8
—	—	—	—	—	★★	2
—	—	—	—	—	—	7
★	—	—	—	—	—	4
—	—	—	—	—	—	0
★	★	—	—	—	—	4

(continued)

All-Star Garden Crops—*continued*

Crop	Protein	Calcium	Phosphorus	Iron
Lettuce, romaine	—	★	—	★
Loganberries	—	—	—	—
Mushrooms	—	—	—	—
Muskmelons	—	—	—	—
Mustard greens	—	★★	—	—
New Zealand spinach	—	—	—	—
Okra	—	★★★	—	—
Onions, dry	—	—	—	—
Onions, green	—	—	—	—
Oranges	—	★	—	—
Peaches	—	—	—	—
Peanuts	★★★★	—	★★★	—
Pears	—	—	—	—
Peas	★	—	—	★
Pecans	—	—	—	—
Peppers, sweet	—	—	—	—
Plums	—	—	—	—
Popcorn	—	—	—	—
Potatoes	★	—	★	—
Radishes	—	—	—	—
Raspberries, black	—	—	—	—
Raspberries, red	—	—	—	—
Rhubarb	—	★	—	—
Rutabagas	—	★	—	—
Salsify	—	—	—	—
Soybeans	★★★★	★	★★★	★★★
Spinach	—	★★	—	★

Potassium	Vitamin A	Thiamine	Riboflavin	Niacin	Vitamin C	Total Stars
★	★	—	—	—	—	4
—	—	—	—	—	—	0
—	—	—	★★★★	★★★★	—	8
★	★	—	—	★	★★	5
—	★	—	★	—	★	5
★★	★	—	—	—	—	3
—	—	★★	★★★	★	—	9
—	—	★★★	—	—	—	3
—	—	—	—	—	—	0
—	—	★	—	—	★★★	5
★	★	—	—	★★	—	4
—	—	★	—	★★★★	—	12
—	—	—	—	—	—	0
—	—	★★★★	★	★★★	★	11
—	—	★★★★	—	—	—	4
—	—	—	—	—	★★★★	4
—	—	—	—	—	—	0
—	—	—	—	—	—	0
★★★★	—	★★	—	★★★★	★	13
—	—	—	—	—	—	0
—	—	—	—	—	—	0
—	—	—	—	—	—	0
—	—	—	—	—	—	1
—	—	—	—	★	★	3
—	—	—	—	—	—	0
★★★	—	★★★	—	—	—	17
—	★★★	—	★	—	★	8

(continued)

All-Star Garden Crops—*continued*

Crop	Protein	Calcium	Phosphorus	Iron
Squash, acorn	—	—	—	—
Squash, butternut	—	—	—	—
Squash, crookneck	—	—	—	—
Squash, Hubbard	—	—	—	—
Squash, scallop	—	—	—	—
Squash, zucchini	—	—	—	—
Strawberries	—	—	—	—
Sunflower seeds	★★★★	—	★★★★	★★★★
Sweet potatoes	—	—	—	—
Tomatoes	—	—	—	—
Turnip greens	—	★★★	—	—
Turnip roots	—	—	—	—
Walnuts, black	★	—	★★★★	★
Walnuts, English	★	—	★	—
Watercress	—	★	—	—
Watermelons	—	—	—	★★
Witloof chicory	—	—	—	—

Superstar Garden Crops

From the preceding chart, All-Star Garden Crops, it's possible to have a little more fun. From these all-star crops can be drawn a list of superstars, those crops that offer the most nutrition in the most categories. Adding up all the stars earned by each crop reveals those that are the overall nutritional powerhouses out of the 89 crops considered.

Just missing the top ten in this ranking is a garden favorite, peas, which may be your best bet for all-around springtime nutrition. Rounding out the rest of the top 20 are avocados, lima beans, great northern beans, kidney beans, okra, watermelons, kale, spinach, butternut squash, sweet

Potassium	Vitamin A	Thiamine	Riboflavin	Niacin	Vitamin C	Total Stars
★★★	—	—	★★	—	—	5
★★★★	★★	—	★★	—	—	8
—	—	—	★	★	—	2
—	★★	—	★★	—	—	4
—	—	—	★	★	—	2
—	—	—	★	★	—	2
—	—	—	—	—	★★	2
★	—	★★★★	—	★★★	—	20
★	★★★★	★	—	★	★	8
★	—	—	—	★	★	3
—	★	★	★★	—	★	8
—	—	—	—	—	★	1
—	—	—	—	—	—	6
—	—	—	—	—	—	2
—	—	—	—	—	★	2
★★	★	★	★	★	★	9
—	—	—	—	—	—	0

potatoes, and turnip greens. (There are actually more than 20 because of a large tie for twentieth place.) These 23 crops, then, may be considered to be the true nutritional superstars of the garden.

Most Nutritionally Versatile Crops

Not content to stop at this, there's yet another way to rank crops for nutrition. Look at navy beans in the preceding superstar rankings, for example. They are tied for sixth place with 14 total stars. They are rich in protein, phosphorus, iron, potassium, and thiamine. But they are not

Superstars: Top Nutritional Star Earners

Ranking	Crop	Stars Earned
1.	Amaranth	24
2.	Sunflower seeds	20
3.	Broccoli	17
(tie)	Soybeans	17
5.	Almonds	15
6.	Collards	14
(tie)	Navy beans	14
8.	Cowpeas	13
(tie)	Potatoes	13
10.	Dandelion greens	12
(tie)	Peanuts	12

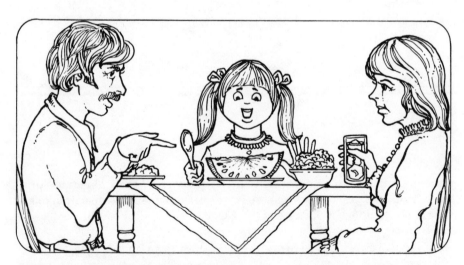

No Spinach Until You Eat Your Watermelon: *This may come as a surprise, but in terms of the number of nutrients they supply, watermelon comes out ahead of spinach. Watermelon is at least an above-average source of seven major nutrients, while spinach supplies only five.*

Most Versatile Garden Crops

Ranking	Crop	Appearances in Ten Categories
1.	Broccoli	9
2.	Amaranth	8
(tie)	Lima beans	8
4.	Cowpeas	7
(tie)	Watermelons	7
6.	Almonds	6
(tie)	Collards	6
(tie)	Peas	6
(tie)	Potatoes	6
(tie)	Soybeans	6
(tie)	Sunflower seeds	6
12.	(a tie among many crops with 5)	

particularly good sources of calcium, vitamin A, riboflavin, niacin, and vitamin C. What if crops were ranked in order of their nutritional versatility, based on the number of areas in which they received at least one star? These would be the crops you could depend on for all-around nutritional performance—nature's version of a multi-vitamin-and-mineral package for the dinner table.

It's interesting to note that, when crops are ranked in this fashion, navy beans do not appear on the list, except in a large tie for twelfth place. But look at which crops do appear on the list. Watermelon is a definite surprise, ranking in seven of ten categories. It is not superlative in any of them, but it is a rich source of iron and potassium and above average in vitamin A, thiamine, riboflavin, niacin, and vitamin C, placing in a tie for fourth place among 89 garden crops. (Spinach, incidentally, is in that large tie for twelfth place. Will enlightened parents now say, "No, you cannot have your spinach until you finish your watermelon!"?)

Putting Rankings in Perspective

Rankings, of course, are not especially meaningful except as bases for broad comparisons. As you know, the nutritional value of any crop varies according to many factors. Still, there are surprises to be found and lessons to be learned.

You might wonder how our all-star listings can be so different from those in the California study mentioned earlier in this chapter, under Vegetables—Capable of So Much More. Asparagus appears nowhere on our lists because it earned only three total stars in the ten nutritional categories. Globe artichokes, fifth in terms of overall nutrient value on the California list, also earned only three stars on ours. Cauliflower got one star, and carrots four (for vitamin A) as compared to a much stronger showing in the California rankings.

One reason for the differences is that the California study ranked only 39 vegetables and fruits, while we ranked 89 vegetables, fruits, and nuts. The California scientists obviously didn't include amaranth as a common garden vegetable. (Amaranth isn't well enough known to be considered common—although we hope it will be, within a few years.) Also, the California study did not consider sunflower seeds and soybeans, which don't appear on popularity charts. But it is difficult to see how that study could have excluded collards, cowpeas, and watermelons, all of which are popular (in some regions more than others) and all of which ranked high on our lists.

Another factor is the measure of the foods used as the basis for analysis. The California study used, as a basis for nutritional rankings, the milligrams of each nutrient present in 100 grams of the food. We converted this same data into average servings: ½ cup cooked spinach, ¼ cup roasted peanuts, a 5-ounce stalk of celery, four medium stalks of asparagus, and so on. There is little point in making pound-for-pound comparisons when we do not eat foods pound for pound. A medium-size potato, weighing 7⅛ ounces, may be said to be an average serving. Four medium spears of asparagus, weighing only 2 ounces, may also be considered an average serving. If we were to compare potatoes and asparagus on a pound-for-pound basis, the asparagus would certainly rise in the nutritional rankings. But we have chosen to compare typical servings because that is how we usually eat these foods. If, at your dinner table, you are used to eating heaps of asparagus and only half a potato, you will of course make adjustments in your evaluations of these crops.

(We have, incidentally, not included in our rankings some garden crops that are used primarily as condiments. These crops don't contribute significantly to our diets even though they may have significant nutritional value on a pound-for-pound basis. Hot chili peppers, for instance, are exceptional sources of vitamin C, offering 778 milligrams in a pound. But you eat chili peppers relatively seldom and in such small amounts that they do not play an important role in your diet. A cup of chopped parsley offers 103 milligrams of vitamin C—but the single sprig that you use to brighten up the dinner plate has less than 1 milligram.)

Better Nutrition from the Garden

How well can your garden feed you? As this chapter points out, very well, indeed. You can get more nutrition from your garden than ever before. You can slant your garden's nutritional production to stress those vitamins and minerals that are most important to you. You can raise crops of higher nutritional value than ever before. And, perhaps most important, you can sharply reduce your dependence on supermarket produce and processed foods of all kinds, raising the quality of your diet to new heights. By now it should be very clear that gardening for nutrition pays rich dividends.

_____ CHAPTER 5 _____

Planning
the Nutrition Garden

If asked to define the criteria for planning the vegetable garden, the average gardener—even one of long experience and considerable skill—would be hard-pressed to answer.

Just how have you planned your own gardens in years past? Of course, you plant those vegetables that you and your family like to eat. Tomatoes are a must. Beans and lettuce are standard. Some gardeners plant squash out of sheer habit. You probably have your own favorite varieties of most vegetables, too. If Kentucky Wonder pole beans have performed well in the past, there's little temptation to change. Nantes carrots are dependable, to the point of becoming sacrosanct in many gardens. And there are some growers who, even though new tomato varieties appear each season, remain faithful to dependable old Rutgers and Beefsteak.

Garden space is another criterion used by most gardeners. The small urban lot must be planned to use every available inch to produce the most vegetables possible. Carrots, onions, bush beans, staked hybrid tomatoes, and peppers are favorite crops since they produce generous amounts in a minimum of space. Potatoes, squash, melons, and sweet corn are usually considered off-limits in small gardens. Vegetable breeders, recognizing the growing interest in small-space gardening, have responded with dwarf varieties of many vegetables and bush forms of cucumbers, squash, and other naturally trailing crops. This expands the selection of vegetables to grow in small spaces.

Gardeners usually give some attention to the winter food supply, as well. The medium-to-large-size garden can supply fresh vegetables from spring to killing frost plus a bonus of surplus crops for canning, freezing, drying, and root cellaring. Large-space gardeners usually plan for a number of good winter keepers including late potatoes, carrots, turnips, and other staples.

The challenge of experimentation and the lure of novelty also figure into the plans of some gardeners. They like to grow a few unusual crops each year, ones that seldom or never appear in their supermarkets. Chinese cabbage, purple-pod bush beans, burpless cucumbers, white eggplants, vegetable spaghetti, and corn salad all turn up from time to time in otherwise prosaic backyard plots. Such forays into the unknown provide a measure of excitement that makes gardening continually interesting.

Sometimes—and more now than in years past—vegetable crops are chosen for their ornamental value. Gardeners have found that parsley makes an attractive edging plant in perennial borders and that the rich green foliage of bell peppers can fit nicely into annual beds. New dwarf vegetable varieties may be tucked into any sunny corner of the home grounds to provide both beauty and food. Breeders are paying close attention to this new interest, too, offering new varieties expressly to serve this dual purpose.

Still, most gardeners never actually define for themselves the criteria they use in choosing crops and varieties. If asked, they probably would think about the question and eventually provide some reasonable answers. But when it actually comes to sitting down with the seed catalogs in January and planning for the coming season, specific criteria seldom come to mind. But if gardeners were forced to list criteria before planning, nutrition would most likely be one of them.

With most gardeners, of course, nutrition is a consideration in garden planning, if only a secondary one. If pressed, the gardener would say that, yes, carrots provide lots of vitamin A. And green peppers are high in vitamin C. And beans provide protein. And spinach is rich in iron—or is it calcium? Beyond a few general impressions, however, most gardeners are ignorant of the specific nutrient attributes of crops. In short, most gardeners have never thought about *planning the garden for nutrition.*

How strange, then, that when asked why they plant vegetables, the same gardeners would answer without hesitation: "To get fresher, better-tasting, and more nutritious food!"

The same gardeners might also be fairly knowledgeable about nutrition needs. They may be aware of the health benefits of selenium but totally unaware that onions are a good source of selenium. They may take vitamin C supplements regularly yet be unaware that they could double their dietary intake of this vitamin merely by growing a different variety of tomato and by growing certain salad greens in place of others, taking absolutely no extra effort, expense, or space in the garden.

The first rule in nutrition-garden planning, then, is to *think nutrition.* Never choose a crop or a variety without considering its nutritional benefits. Think of your home food supply and your nutrition needs as two sides of a single coin. By doing so, you will raise the quality of your garden to one of a dependable and high-powered nutrition factory. Planning is the key.

What must you give up to plan and plant your garden nutritionally? Nothing. You can still plant all the vegetables you love, and you can hold onto the varieties you have come to depend on and treasure. You can satisfy your need for gardening adventure, and your garden can be just as beautiful as ever. You will find yourself planting more of some vegetables than others, searching the catalogs for special varieties, and trying some crops that you have never tried before. You will make adjustments slowly or en masse, as you choose. And you will soon find that you are automatically paying more attention than ever to your dietary needs. You will know

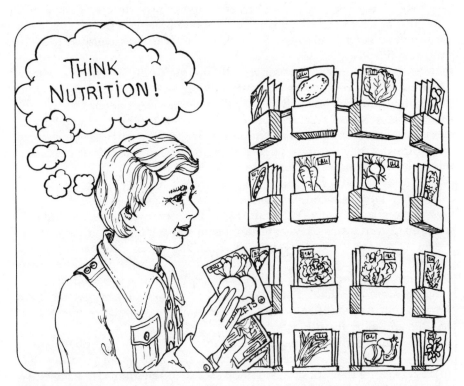

The First Rule in Planning: *As you select your garden crops, always consider their nutritional benefits.*

which vitamins and minerals are not being supplied adequately by your daily diet, and you will then be able to supplement those needs in a fully informed way.

Optimum Nutrition from the Garden

Your goal is to supply as many of your nutritional needs as you can from the garden space available. Ideally, a family of four can supply nearly all of their nutritional needs on a half acre of land, with proper selection of crops and the use of intensive gardening techniques.

Most likely, however, total self-sufficiency will not be your goal. Perhaps you merely want to improve the nutritional capacity of the garden you now have. Or you might want to enlarge the garden and improve your methods to gain a sharp increase in your supply of dependable, pesticide-free, fresh garden produce. But it is both reassuring and inspiring to realize that a medium-to-large-size garden, when modern organic methods are used, is capable of supplying total nutritional needs. Your efforts can, and should, be geared to fit your individual needs and lifestyle.

Selecting Crops

Your knowledge of a balanced diet will be your key to planning a nutritionally balanced garden. If you are more diet- and health-conscious than most people, you can easily apply your special knowledge to planning the garden for your specific nutrition needs. If your interest in nutrition is not quite so keen, then you may simply want to include in the garden a well-rounded selection of crops that, together, supply good amounts of all the major nutrients. To streamline your planning, use the box Some Garden Sources of Major Nutrients as a starting point in selecting crops for your nutrition garden.

Four Rules of Planning for Nutrition

• Select a range of crops and specific varieties of crops to supply the widest variety and greatest amounts of all the essential vitamins and minerals.
• Adopt organic soil-building practices to assure the highest reasonable level of naturally occurring minerals and other nutrients which are transferred to food portions of crops.
• Learn to get the most food from a given area of garden space, using both intensive gardening techniques and season-stretching methods.
• Store and prepare foods for the table in ways that will preserve the greatest amounts of vitamins and minerals.

Some Garden Sources of Major Nutrients

For vitamin A: carrots, collards, leafy greens, orange-fleshed squash, sweet potatoes

For thiamine (vitamin B₁): beans, cowpeas, okra, onions, peas, pecans, potatoes, soybeans, sunflower seeds

For riboflavin (vitamin B₂): almonds, avocados, broccoli, collards, leafy greens, mushrooms, okra, winter squash

For niacin (vitamin B₃): amaranth, avocados, cowpeas, mushrooms, peaches, peanuts, peas, potatoes, sunflower seeds

For vitamin C: amaranth, broccoli, Brussels sprouts, cabbage, citrus fruits, collards, kale, kohlrabi, muskmelons, sweet peppers, strawberries

For potassium: amaranth, avocados, beans, New Zealand spinach, potatoes, soybeans, squash, watermelons

For phosphorus: beans, cowpeas, lentils, nuts, soybeans, sunflower seeds

For calcium: almonds, amaranth, broccoli, collards, leafy greens, okra

For protein: almonds, beans, cowpeas, lentils, peanuts, soybeans, sunflower seeds

For iron: amaranth, beans, lentils, butterhead lettuce, soybeans, sunflower seeds, watermelons

For fiber: almonds, apples, beans, corn, peas, plums, potatoes, spinach, sweet potatoes

Of course, there are other elements necessary to total nutrition in addition to those covered in the box. These include trace elements such as magnesium, copper, manganese, and selenium. Sufficient amounts of each will be present in a wide variety of vegetables, and their presence in your garden crops will depend to a significant degree on your soil-building practices, as discussed earlier in chapter 3.

In addition to nutritional considerations, you should also base your crop selection on such factors as whether the climate in your area is favorable, whether your season is long enough for the crop to mature, and whether you can meet its basic cultural needs. Chapter 7 provides a rundown of this information for 76 fruits, vegetables, and nuts to help you make your decision on what to grow in the nutrition garden.

You will note, in going over the crop recommendations throughout this book, the frequent appearance of certain vegetables such as amaranth, dried beans, broccoli, cowpeas, sunflower seeds, and others. These are truly the nutrition stars of the garden, deserving increased attention among gardeners everywhere. Beans for drying are especially valuable, offering significant amounts of protein, B-complex vitamins, potassium,

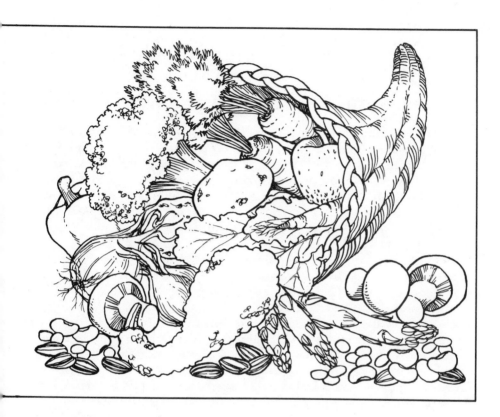

phosphorus, and fiber—and yet they are not among the more popular of garden crops. In the nutrition garden, they should be well represented. And even those gardeners who choose not to plant some of them, possibly for reasons of space limitations or a too-short growing season, should still buy them in dried form and use them more often in the daily diet. By knowing how much nutrition your garden can supply, you will also know what foods you need as supplements to garden nutrition.

How about some favorite garden crops that appear seldom—or not at all—in the high-nutrition lists? What's the status of tomatoes, apples, celery, green beans, beets, and radishes in the nutrition garden? Even though they may not shine in various nutritional areas, they're worth growing because they contain modest amounts of a broad variety of nutrients and because they offer dietary variety. Tomatoes are a prime example. They are a good (but not spectacular) source of vitamin C, containing 28 milligrams in one fresh, medium-sized (4¾ ounces) fruit, which is 47 percent of the Adult Recommended Dietary Allowance (R.D.A.). That same tomato provides 1,110 International Units of vitamin A (22 percent of the R.D.A.) and lesser amounts of 18 other vitamins and minerals as well. Beet roots, which look so meaty and nutritious, unfortunately are a poor vitamin and mineral package. Nutritionally speaking, you would do well to focus on the greens and throw away the roots—except that they taste so good.

Variations in Vitamins and Minerals

It would be nice if you could plan your vegetable garden down to the last milligram of vitamin C or the final International Unit of vitamin A. If that were the case, you could spend your time in such absorbing calculations as these: a 1-foot row of carrots will produce ten large roots; at 11,000 International Units each, that's 110,000 total International Units, or enough vitamin A for 22 days for one adult; there are four people in the family, 365 days in the year . . . and so on and so forth.

Unfortunately (or perhaps fortunately), even those of us who enjoy fine mathematical projections would be wasting our time in applying the effort to this purpose. The process simply cannot be carried to this fine a point for two reasons. First, the size of the crop will vary according to soil, weather, and all the other garden conditions that make for good and bad years. Second, the official vitamin and mineral charts prepared by the United States Department of Agriculture (USDA) are not fully reliable. Indeed, they are sometimes grossly inaccurate since they rely on a worldwide search of studies for data rather than on their own analysis. A few years ago, Consumers Union (C.U.) compared their own test results on Russet Burbank potatoes to the USDA figures. Whereas the USDA showed a medium-size potato to contain 20 milligrams of vitamin C, the C.U. tests showed only 5 milligrams. That's quite a difference. Moreover, the quality of the potato's protein was found to be much poorer than previously thought. United Nations figures rate the protein in a potato as being 71 percent as efficient as the protein in an egg (the egg being considered perfect protein). The C.U. tests, however, pegged the potato's protein efficiency at only 17 percent, indicating that commercially grown potatoes (these were bought in a supermarket) may in fact be a poor source of protein for human needs. As it was discussed in chapter 3, the vitamin and mineral content of vegetables and fruits can be affected greatly by the soil in which they are grown. This is one big reason for growing as much of your own food as possible—but also a reason why you can't depend fully on the official nutrition charts. Your garden planning can serve as a broad gauge of the nutritional return you may expect—but it cannot accurately project milligrams, calories, and International Units.

A sound plan of action will assure that your own garden crops have maximum nutritional value. First, choose the most nutritious crops and varieties, then build your soil to the greatest possible level of richness, and finally, use those harvesting, storing, and kitchen preparation methods that will preserve the greatest level of nutrition in every crop. Chapters 2, 3, and 7 give you the tools you need to achieve each of these three goals.

Substituting Crops for Better Nutrition

By substituting just a few crops for others and by diversifying your plantings (growing a greater number of crops but less of some than others), you can raise the total nutrition yield of your garden dramatically without increasing its size. And you can hold onto your favorite crops and trusted varieties even if they are not overly rich in nutritional value.

As an example, take a look at an early spring garden in a northern temperate region. This sample garden contains only a few standard crops, which are planted as early in the season as possible and harvested in less than 50 days. In past years, this part of the garden has included the standard leaf lettuce, radishes, spinach, and onions. (In fact, your spring garden will probably contain more than this, but for purposes of comparison this garden will be limited to these four crops.)

Now, after studying the nutrient charts, a change in the crop selection is in order. Radishes and onions are eliminated, and turnips and beets are planted in their place. The turnips and beets will be used for their greens, and their roots will be—nutritionally speaking—a minor bonus.

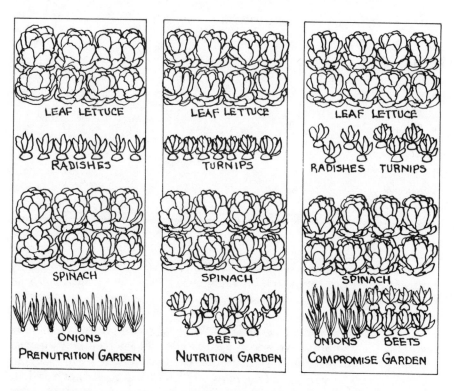

Early Spring Garden: *These three views of the same garden should give you some idea of how easy it is to raise the nutritional yield of the garden without enlarging it.*

The Early Spring Garden

	Vitamin A (I.U.)	Vitamin C (mg)	Calcium (mg)	Iron (mg)
Standard Garden				
Leaf lettuce (4 oz.)	2,155	21	77	1.6
Radishes (5 med.)	trace	6	7	0.3
Spinach (½ cup, cooked)	7,290	25	84	2.0
Onion (2 oz., green)	1,134	18	29	0.6
Averages	2,645	17.5	49	1.13
Nutrition Garden				
Spinach (½ cup, cooked)	7,290	25	84	2.0
Leaf lettuce (4 oz.)	2,155	21	77	1.6
Beet greens (½ cup, cooked)	3,700	11	72	1.4
Turnip greens (½ cup, cooked)	4,135	34	126	0.8
Averages	4,320	23	90	1.45

This doesn't seem like much of a change—hardly a revolution in the early spring garden. But you'll probably be surprised to see what happens when the two plans are compared in terms of some representative vitamins and minerals.

Something as simple as making these two crop substitutions has increased the vitamin A average by approximately 63 percent, the vitamin C average by 31 percent, the calcium by 84 percent, and the iron by 28 percent, based on average serving portions. (Comparisons are not based on yield per square foot in the garden; it seems more reasonable to judge the food right on the dinner table, where it affects health most directly.) At the same time, there's been no increase in garden space, expense, or effort—and there are some beet and turnip roots as a tasty bonus. This nutritional rise in stature is due to the fact that two nutritional powerhouses—beet greens and turnip greens—were substituted for onions and radishes. (Radishes, in particular, are nutritional lightweights.)

But what if you don't want to give up radishes and onions? Certainly they do add zest to springtime salads. The fact is, you don't have to give them up. You can go ahead and include them in the nutritional garden but at the same time reduce the amounts of all crops so that you plant no more row feet in total. This way you'll still increase the nutritional yield of the garden while holding onto the crops dearest to your heart. You will have created a compromise garden, which is a very important concept when you are trying to raise the household nutritional level while preserving harmony.

The example of the springtime garden may be repeated for different periods of the growing season and in different climates. Just for fun, take a look at some representative crops that might be found in a midsummer garden in a warm climate. Assume that the garden will contain tomatoes, okra, sweet corn, green snap beans, cucumbers, zucchini squash, watermelons, Brussels sprouts, eggplants, and cauliflower, all commonly grown vegetables. By referring back to the nutritional charts in chapter 4, it's easy to plan how to upgrade this garden's nutritional yield. Based on their relative nutritional merits, cucumbers, zucchini, green snap beans, Brussels sprouts, cauliflower, and eggplants are dropped, and collards, sweet potatoes, amaranth, cowpeas, green peppers, and broccoli are substituted. The tomatoes, sweet corn, okra, and watermelons will stay because summer just wouldn't be summer without them. The following chart shows what happens when these changes in the garden lineup are made.

As you can see from the averages, the yield of vitamin A has been increased by 455 percent, thiamine by 57 percent, vitamin C by 114 percent, calcium by 193 percent, and iron by 86 percent. Again, it's quite clear that when you select crops with nutrition in mind, you can make a sizable difference in your garden's nutritional profile.

But what if some household members protest the elimination of favorite vegetables, those squeezed out of the garden because they came up light on the nutrition charts? The answer is that they don't have to be squeezed out at all. Eating, after all, should be enjoyable as well as nutritious, and accommodations can always be made. To demonstrate, just think back to the principle of the compromise garden. Say that, originally, you had planned to plant one row each of tomatoes, okra, sweet corn, green snap beans, eggplants, cucumbers, zucchini, watermelons, Brussels sprouts, and cauliflower. In order to increase the total nutritional yield, you eliminated six of these, much to the dismay of those in the family who love these vegetables. A good compromise would be to plant a full row

(continued on page 93)

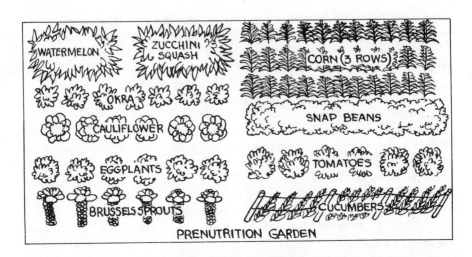

PRENUTRITION GARDEN

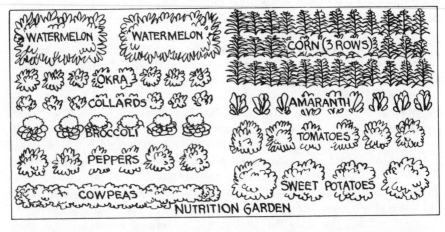

NUTRITION GARDEN

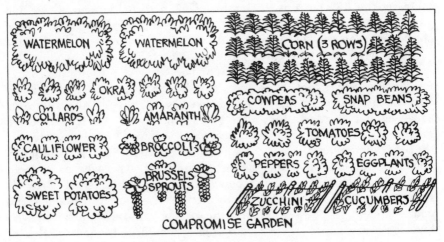

COMPROMISE GARDEN

Midsummer Garden: *Substituting certain crops for others and diversifying the plantings are keys to boosting the garden's nutritional yield. The views at left of the same garden planted with three different sets of crops can serve as examples for you to follow in your own garden planning.*

The Summer Garden

	Vitamin A (I.U.)	Thiamine (mg)	Vitamin C (mg)	Calcium (mg)	Iron (mg)
Standard Garden					
Cucumber (½ cup, sliced)	130	0.02	6	13	0.6
Zucchini squash (½ cup, cooked)	360	0.06	11	30	0.5
Tomato (1 med., raw)	1,100	0.07	28	16	0.6
Sweet corn (½ cup, cooked)	330	0.09	6	3	0.5
Green snap beans (½ cup, cooked)	340	0.04	7	32	0.4
Eggplant (½ cup, cooked)	10	0.05	3	11	0.6
Okra (4 oz., cooked)	555	0.15	23	104	0.6
Watermelon (1-in.-thick, 10-in.-diameter slice)	2,510	0.13	30	30	2.1
Brussels sprouts (4 sprouts, cooked)	405	0.06	68	25	0.9
Cauliflower (½ cup, cooked)	40	0.06	35	13	0.5
Averages	578	0.07	22	28	0.7
Nutrition Garden					
Amaranth (4 oz., raw)	6,918	0.09	91	303	4.4

(continued)

The Summer Garden — *continued*

	Vitamin A (I.U.)	Thiamine (mg)	Vitamin C (mg)	Calcium (mg)	Iron (mg)
Nutrition Garden — *continued*					
Tomato (1 med., raw)	1,100	0.07	28	16	0.6
Sweet corn (½ cup, cooked)	330	0.09	6	3	0.5
Cowpeas (½ cup, cooked)	290	0.25	14	20	1.8
Sweet potato (1 med., baked)	9,230	0.10	25	46	1.0
Collards (½ cup, cooked)	7,410	0.07	49	168	0.8
Okra (4 oz., cooked)	555	0.15	23	104	0.6
Sweet pepper (1 med., raw)	244	0.05	74	6	0.4
Broccoli (1 sm. stalk, cooked)	3,500	0.13	126	123	1.1
Watermelon (1-in.-thick, 10-in.-diameter slice)	2,510	0.13	30	30	2.1
Averages	3,209	0.11	47	82	1.3
Compromise Garden					
Tomato (1 med., raw)	1,100	0.07	28	16	0.6
Sweet corn (½ cup, cooked)	330	0.09	6	3	0.5
Okra (4 oz., cooked)	555	0.15	23	104	0.6
Watermelon (1-in.-thick, 10-in.-diameter slice)	2,510	0.13	30	30	2.1
Green snap beans* (¼ cup, cooked)	170	0.02	4	16	0.2

	Vitamin A (I.U.)	Thiamine (mg)	Vitamin C (mg)	Calcium (mg)	Iron (mg)
Eggplant* (¼ cup, cooked)	5	0.03	2	6	0.3
Cucumber* (¼ cup, sliced)	65	0.01	3	7	0.3
Zucchini squash (¼ cup, cooked)	180	0.03	6	15	0.3
Brussels sprouts* (2 sprouts, cooked)	203	0.03	34	13	0.5
Cauliflower* (¼ cup, cooked)	20	0.03	18	7	0.3
Collards* (¼ cup, cooked)	3,705	0.04	25	84	0.4
Sweet potato* (½ med., baked)	4,615	0.05	13	23	0.5
Amaranth* (2 oz., raw)	3,459	0.05	46	152	2.2
Cowpeas* (¼ cup, cooked)	145	0.13	7	10	0.9
Sweet pepper* (½ med., raw)	122	0.03	37	3	0.2
Broccoli* (½ sm. stalk, cooked)	1,750	0.07	63	62	0.6
Averages	1,893	0.10	35	55	1.1

*Each counts ½ serving (corresponding to ½ row planted) when computing averages.

each of tomatoes, sweet corn, okra, and watermelons and a half row each of green snap beans, eggplants, collards, sweet potatoes, amaranth, cowpeas, peppers, broccoli, cucumbers, zucchini, Brussels sprouts, and cauliflower. You will now have a garden of wider crop variety with a full complement of the "must" crops and reduced plantings of all the others. You're still planting ten rows. And when you compare the nutritional yield of this compromise garden with that of the original garden, you'll still find a healthy nutritional improvement.

If you compare the nutrient averages of the compromise garden with those of the standard summer garden, you still find vitamin A yield increasing by 228 percent and thiamine by 43 percent, vitamin C by 59 percent, calcium by 96 percent, and iron by 57 percent. These figures tell you that you don't have to sacrifice the crops you love in the pursuit of higher nutrition from the garden.

Now, just how meaningful are these comparisons? Obviously, you can't compare a cup of cooked cauliflower to a row of collards or a bushel of tomatoes to a half cup of cowpeas. But these figures are valuable as general sources of comparison. By studying these comparisons, you can certainly conclude that a 50-foot row of amaranth will yield greater total nutrition than a 50-foot row of cucumbers. You can see that broccoli has ten times as much vitamin A as snap beans. And you can see that, if you're trying to add more calcium to your diet, sweet corn isn't going to do much for you, but collards will. Perhaps this year you will want to try amaranth for the first time. You might decide to plant more broccoli and fewer snap beans. And if there is a growing child in the house, you might want to introduce more of the calcium-rich vegetables. These one-on-one comparisons are valuable for these purposes. But they don't tell you the whole story. There are some other factors that are important in planning the nutrition garden.

Yield per square foot of gardening space: If you are looking for an optimum amount of vitamin A from a given area of garden, you may note that ½ cup of cooked collards provides roughly 7,410 International Units of A while one sweet potato (which weighs the same) provides an average of 9,230 International Units. Before you choose in favor of the sweet potato, consider the yields of each. From one row foot you might get three or four potatoes but somewhere around 10 cups of edible collard leaves. When judged on this basis, that garden space might yield more total vitamin A if planted to collards. Or you might decide to compromise and plant both. Yield is certainly a factor to consider, especially if gardening space is limited.

Days to harvest: Again, when considering total nutritional harvest from a given area, you must take into account the length of time to maturity for each crop. Even though, for instance, garden cress has somewhat less calcium than okra, you can grow three to five crops of cress in the time it takes to produce a single crop of okra. And even though Hubbard squash may provide copious amounts of vitamin A, it does occupy its space in the garden for most or all of the season. Perhaps a series of two or three faster-growing succession crops might make better use of that space if your garden area is limited. Also take into account the season-length limitations

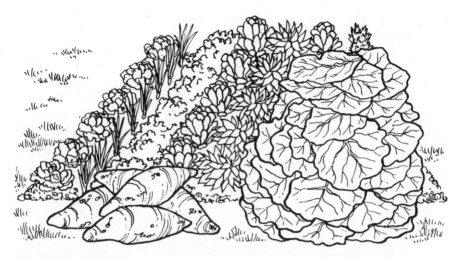

Consider the Yield: *When judging which crops to include in the nutrition garden, don't forget to take yield into account. For example, sweet potatoes and collards are both very good sources of vitamin A. To get the most vitamin A out of a foot of garden row, you'd be better off planting the collards, since you'll harvest ten cups of leaves versus only three or four sweet potatoes.*

of your climate. For some northern gardeners, there just may not be enough time to raise a crop of sweet potatoes or dry beans to maturity. Chapter 7 gives the time to harvest for 76 fruit, vegetable, and nut crops, so you can see at a glance whether a particular crop is suitable for your area.

Average edible portion: It's impressive to consider that a single cup of hot chili peppers contains 23,500 International Units of vitamin A—until you stop and think about eating a cup of hot chili peppers. Consider the portions of various foods that will actually be eaten at the table. Potatoes and beans, for instance, will count for more than onions and peppers because you usually eat greater quantities of the former at a typical meal. Consider also the frequency with which you eat certain foods. Again, potatoes and beans are likely to appear more often on the household menu than eggplant and Brussels sprouts.

The total diet: Unless you are a vegetarian living completely off the land, major portions of certain vitamins and minerals will come from foods other than your homegrown vegetables and fruits. You may depend largely on eggs and dairy products for your daily protein allowance, so protein yield may not be your prime consideration in planning the vegetable garden. (If, on the other hand, you *are* a vegetarian, then it will be a major concern.) For your supply of thiamine, you may find it more convenient to depend primarily on liver or nutritional yeast than on garden vegetables, which seldom offer large amounts of this nutrient. Consider your entire diet when placing values on garden crops.

In addition, your garden crop selections should take into account your actual and total dietary needs. If you decide that you would like to keep your vitamin A intake at around 10,000 International Units a day, then there would not be much point in overloading the garden—or your table—with this vitamin. A single meal of roast chicken, collards, and a sweet potato will give you more than 17,000 International Units of A. Add a quarter of a cantaloupe for dessert, and you will have doubled your planned intake at a single sitting. The philosophy of nutritional variety and balance should be practiced in the garden and carried through to the dinner table.

Getting the Most Out of the Row

For limited-space gardeners, especially, intensive gardening techniques are important for getting the most out of every row. Perhaps you already use succession planting, intercropping, relay planting, wide-row planting, and double-row planting to boost the total crop yield from your garden. Now you can use these methods to get more total nutrition from each and every row. This section will be only a brief review of these intensive gardening techniques since the methods are well covered in other books (see Recommended Reading).

Succession planting: When you make succession plantings you follow an early crop with a later one in the same space. After the spring peas are harvested, you can use that space to grow late cabbage, tomatoes, or eggplants. Spinach can be followed by carrots, cauliflower by Chinese cabbage, radishes by cucumbers, spinach by tomatoes. Even if you garden in a relatively short-season area, you can often raise three crops in the same row. All it takes is careful planning. Be sure to pay attention to the nutrient needs of the succession crops and the days to harvest of each.

Intercropping: With this technique you are planting more than a single crop in the same space. The trick is to make sure compatible crops are sharing the space at the same time. Deep-rooted crops get along well with shallow-rooted ones, since both crops can occupy the same space with no root competition. Tuck compact crops such as radishes, beets, parsley, and onions in with taller-growing tomatoes, broccoli, and Brussels sprouts. This way, they require no rows of their own. You can sow radishes with carrots and then harvest them before the slower-growing carrots need the room to expand. Onions may be interplanted with a number of crops and can be harvested as scallions before the companion crops reach appreciable size. Intercropping is a good way to gain extra nutritional yields by sharing space.

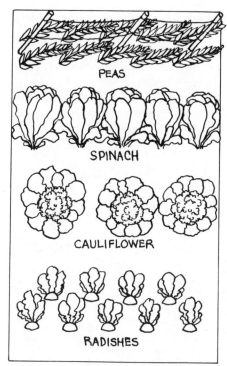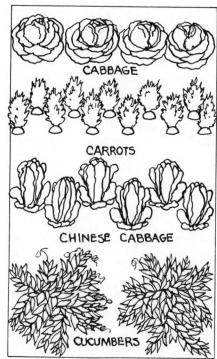

Succession Planting: *As soon as one crop is harvested, plan to fill the empty space with a second crop. Here, cabbage fills in for peas, carrots follow spinach, Chinese cabbage replaces cauliflower, and cucumbers take the place of radishes.*

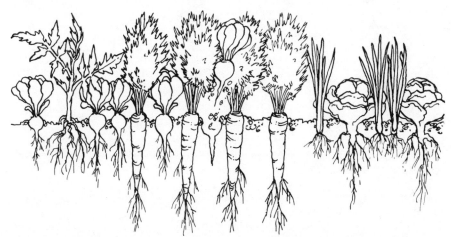

Interplanting: *Make the same garden space do double duty by planting compatible crops close together. Here, radishes nestle around a tomato seedling. The mature roots will be harvested by the time the seedling starts to fill out. Young carrots and ready-to-harvest radishes share cozy quarters for now; the harvested radishes will make way for the expanding carrots. Scallions flourish among young cabbage heads; by the time the cabbages need more growing room, the scallions will have been pulled up for kitchen use.*

Relay planting: This is simply a variation of succession planting in which a single crop is sown a number of times, the sowings separated by a week or so. The three crops most commonly relayed are green snap beans, leaf lettuce, and sweet corn, although the method may be used also for radishes, green onions, and potatoes. The effect is to spread the harvest of these crops over a longer period of time. Instead of harvesting all your sweet corn during a two-week period, you will have a continuing supply for fresh table use over a six- or seven-week period. Relay planting, in itself, will not increase total nutritional yield, although you can use it in

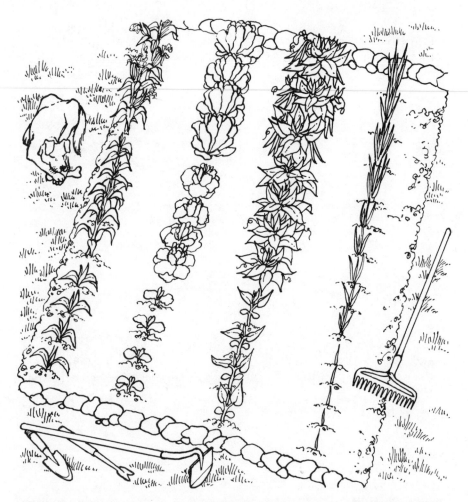

Relay Planting: *Staggered plantings of crops like corn, leaf lettuce, snap beans, and scallions won't hit you with a glut of ripe produce all at once. A staggered harvest, besides being more convenient, is also a good way to ensure a steady stream of garden-fresh nutrients.*

conjunction with succession planting to boost total production. If your sweet corn is traditionally planted on May 1, for instance, and you reserve part of the corn patch for a third relay planting on May 22, then you may use that reserved area for a longer-growing spring crop, one that will reach maturity just before the final relay of corn is sown.

Wide-row planting: This technique is capable of producing up to four times the yield of conventional single-row plantings of certain crops. The usual width of a wide row is 18 inches, with the rows spaced 24 to 30 inches apart. Seed is scattered throughout the wide row instead of being dribbled down single rows. This means the plants are more crowded as they mature. Yields are less per plant but much greater per square foot of space occupied. Good candidates for wide-row planting are bush beans, beets, onions, radishes, parsley, carrots, and other leafy and compact crops.

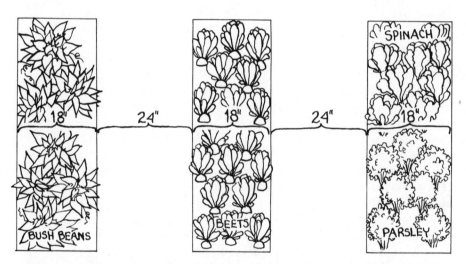

Wide-Row Planting: *You can get four times more yield from a wide row than you would from a conventional single row. Wide rows usually measure 18 inches across, with 24 to 30 inches between rows. Seed is broadcast across the row instead of being lined up precisely, in single file.*

Double-row planting: This is nothing more than a modification of wide-row planting. Instead of a broad band or row, two ordinary rows of the crop are planted very close together, with the normal spacing allowed between each of the double rows. Carrots, for instance, which usually need 15 to 18 inches between single rows, would be planted in double rows only 3 inches apart, each double row spaced 15 to 18 inches from the other. The carrot yield will be increased easily by two-thirds, with the usual amount of room left between rows to work among the plants.

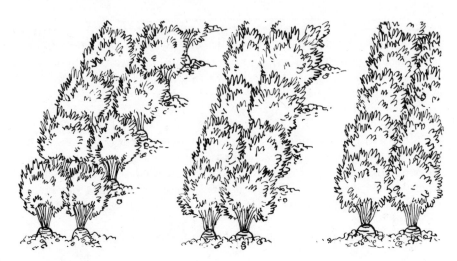

Double-Row Planting: *This intensive method makes better use of garden space than the more conventional single-row method.*

All of these intensive methods rely on a single principle—allow as little of your garden space as possible to lie idle during any time of the growing season. Even when the potato vines die down, a week or two before the first frost, there is still time to squeeze in a good crop of garden cress, rich in vitamins A and C, for fresh use and for freezing. Just cut away the dead potato vines, remove the mulch between the rows, and broadcast as much cress seed as you can. Harvest it all before the first hard freeze of autumn for an extra bonus of important vitamins—in a space and at a time you may never have used before.

Planning for Nutritional Balance

In addition to planning for maximum crop and total nutritional yield, you must pay close attention to nutritional *balance* throughout the gardening season. It would not serve your goals to harvest the bulk of your C-rich crops in the spring, then the C-poor crops in late summer. Nor would it be a good idea to have a bumper crop of vitamin A-rich vegetables in August, but to lack them in the spring. Your goal is to have a full complement of balanced nutrition coming from the garden throughout the entire season, with enough surplus to put up for winter use. This isn't difficult in any climate, but it does take careful planning.

In chapter 4, the all-star crops were introduced, those crops from each of ten nutritional areas that rank above all others. This listing of nutritional winners can help you create garden plans for year-round nutritional balance. The Crop Selection Guide that follows lists eight nutritional areas:

Crop Selection Guide: High-Level Nutrition throughout the Season

For Protein

Early-Season Crop
  Peas★
Mid- to Late-Season Crops
  Lima beans★★
  Cowpeas★★
  Potatoes★
Late-Season Crops
  Kidney beans★★★
  Lentils★★★
  Peanuts★★★★
  Soybeans★★★★
  Sunflower seeds★★★★
Optional Crop
  Almonds★★

For Calcium

Early-Season Crops
  Dandelion greens★★★★
  Spinach★★
  Turnip greens★★★
Mid- to Late-Season Crops
  Amaranth★★★★
  Broccoli★★★
  Collards★★★★
  Honeydew melons★★
  Kale★★
  Okra★★★
Optional Crop
  Almonds★★

For Phosphorus

Mid- to Late-Season Crops
  Lima beans★
  Broccoli★
  Cowpeas★★
  Potatoes★
Late-Season Crops
  Great northern beans★★
  Kidney beans★★
  Navy beans★★★
  Peanuts★★★
  Soybeans★★★
  Sunflower seeds★★★★
Optional Crops
  Almonds★★★★
  Black walnuts★★★★
  English walnuts★

For Vitamin A

Early-Season Crops
  Beet greens★
  Dandelion greens★★★★
  Garden cress★★
  Spinach★★★
Mid- to Late-Season Crops
  Amaranth★★★
  Carrots★★★★
  Collards★★★
  Caro-Rich tomatoes★★
  Chard★★

(continued)

★★★★ Exceptionally rich source ★★ Rich source

★★★ Very rich source ★ Above-average source

Crop Selection Guide—*continued*

For Vitamin A — *continued*
  Late-Season Crops
    Sweet potatoes★★★★
    Butternut squash★★
    Hubbard squash★★

For Potassium
  Early-Season Crops
    Butterhead lettuce★
    Leaf lettuce★
    Romaine lettuce★
  Mid- to Late-Season Crops
    Amaranth★★★
    New Zealand spinach★★
    Potatoes★★★★
    Watermelons★★
  Late-Season Crops
    Great northern beans★★
    Navy beans★★
    Soybeans★★★
    Acorn squash★★★
    Butternut squash★★★★
  Optional Crop
    Avocados★★★★

For Iron
  Early-Season Crops
    Butterhead lettuce★★
    Romaine lettuce★
    Peas★
    Spinach★
  Mid- to Late-Season Crops
    Amaranth★★★★
    Lima beans★★
    Cowpeas★

Late-Season Crops
  Great northern beans★★★
  Kidney beans★★
  Navy beans★★★★
  Soybeans★★★
  Sunflower seeds★★★★

For the Vitamin B Complex
  Early-Season Crops
    Dandelion greens (B_1)★ (B_2)★★
    Peas (B_1)★★★★ (B_3)★★★
    Turnip greens (B_1)★ (B_2)★★
  Mid- to Late-Season Crops
    Amaranth (B_2)★★★ (B_3)★★
    Lima beans (B_1)★★
    Broccoli (B_2)★★★★
    Collards (B_2)★★
    Cowpeas (B_1)★★★★ (B_3)★★
    Okra (B_1)★★ (B_2)★★★
    Onions, dry (B_1)★★★
    Potatoes (B_1)★★ (B_3)★★★★
  Late-Season Crops
    Navy beans (B_1)★★
    Peanuts (B_3)★★★★
    Soybeans (B_1)★★★
    Acorn squash (B_2)★★
    Butternut squash (B_2)★★
    Hubbard squash (B_2)★★
    Sunflower seeds (B_1)★★★★
    (B_3)★★★
  Optional Crops
    Almonds (B_2)★★★★ (B_3)★★
    Avocados (B_2)★★★ (B_3)★★★
    Mushrooms (B_2)★★★★ (B_3)★★★★
    Peaches (B_3)★★
    Pecans (B_1)★★★

For Vitamin C

   Early-Season Crops

      Peas★

      Spinach★

      Strawberries★★

   Mid- to Late-Season Crops

      Amaranth★★★★

      Broccoli★★★★

      Brussels sprouts★★★

      Cabbage★★

      Collards★★★

      Kale★★★

      Kohlrabi★★

      Muskmelons★★

      Sweet peppers★★★★

      Doublerich tomatoes★★

   Optional Crops

      Oranges★★★

      Grapefruit★★

protein, calcium, phosphorus, iron, potassium, vitamin A, the vitamin B complex, and vitamin C. Under each nutritional area, the best garden sources are given, taken from chapter 4's listing of all-star crops. These fruits, vegetables, and nuts are broken down into early-season, mid- to late-season, and late-season harvesting times. Also included are some valuable optional crops that can't be grown in most temperate zones but may be an option for gardeners in favorable climates.

Using this chart, you can make your own season-long garden plan, using the principles of succession planting and intercropping, to create nutritionally balanced harvests that stretch from spring through autumn frost. You will notice that some crops shine in several areas, and it's these crops that you can count on to serve double or triple duty in your nutritional plan.

The Crop Selection Guide can also come in handy as you make your plans for winter crop storage, whether by root cellaring, freezing, canning, or drying. Calculating the needs of the household, you can grow and preserve enough to carry you over to the following season's spring harvests. More about this in chapter 6, which gives tips on nutrient-preserving harvest and storage techniques.

How Much Will the Garden Yield?

The point was made earlier that you cannot calculate the annual household need for each milligram of vitamin C, then plan your garden to provide exactly that total. There are too many variables in crop yields, crop varieties, and even in individual human needs to make this anything other than a futile quest.

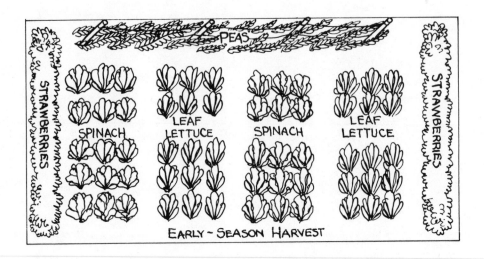

EARLY~SEASON HARVEST

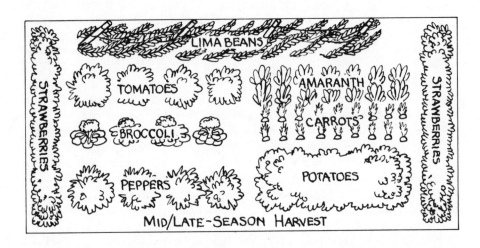

MID/LATE-SEASON HARVEST

Nevertheless, you should have some idea of how much of a yield you can expect from the crops you grow. The chart Estimated Vegetable and Fruit Yields tells you how much you'll harvest from a 100-foot row based on average yields of various crops. Integrating this information with your plans for succession planting and intercropping, you can gain a good idea of how much of each crop you can harvest from your garden for fresh use, preserving, and storing. To help you further with your planning, the charts Approximate Yield of Frozen Produce from Fresh and Approximate Yield of Canned Produce from Fresh will help you figure how much fresh produce you'll need in order to preserve enough to see your family through the winter.

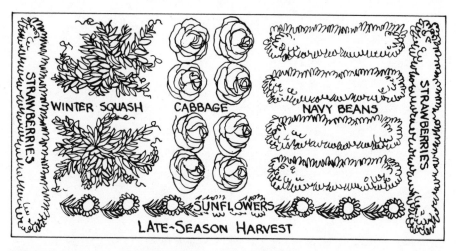

Three Seasons in a Nutrition Garden: *Here's an example of the nutritional contributions a garden can make. In the early-season harvest shown at top left, peas supply protein, iron, B vitamins, vitamin C; spinach supplies calcium, iron, vitamin A; leaf lettuce supplies potassium; and strawberries supply vitamin C. Missing from the harvest is phosphorus; last year's stored dry beans can supplement fresh garden produce at this point in the season. In the mid/late-season harvest shown at bottom left, lima beans provide protein, phosphorus, iron, thiamine; amaranth provides calcium, iron, potassium, vitamin A, riboflavin, vitamin B_3, vitamin C; broccoli provides calcium, phosphorus, riboflavin, vitamin C; potatoes provide phosphorus, potassium, thiamine, vitamin B_3; Caro-Rich tomatoes and carrots provide vitamin A; sweet peppers provide vitamin C. In the late-season harvest shown above (some of which can be carried over in winter storage), navy beans offer protein, phosphorus, iron, potassium, thiamine; sunflower seeds offer protein, phosphorus, iron, thiamine, riboflavin; winter squash offers potassium, vitamin A, riboflavin; late cabbage offers vitamin C.*

Estimated Vegetable and Fruit Yields

Vegetables	Yield per 100 Feet of Row	Vegetables	Yield per 100 Feet of Row
Amaranth	80–100 lb.	Beans, pole snap	150 lb.
Asparagus	30 lb.	Beet roots	150 lb.
Beans, dry	100 lb.	Broccoli	100 lb.
Beans, bush lima	25 lb.	Brussels sprouts	75 lb.
Beans, pole lima	50 lb.	Cabbage	150 lb.
Beans, bush snap	120 lb.	Carrots	100 lb.

(continued)

Vegetables	Yield per 100 Feet of Row	Vegetables	Yield per 100 Feet of Row
Cauliflower	100 lb.	Peanuts	30–50 lb.
Celeriac	60 lb.	Peas	30 lb.
Celery	180 stalks	Peppers, sweet	60 lb.
Chard	40–75 lb.	Potatoes	100 lb.
Chinese cabbage	100 lb.	Pumpkins	300 lb.
Collards	33–150 lb.	Radishes	40 lb.
Corn	120 ears	Rhubarb	180 lb.
Corn salad	25–35 lb.	Rutabagas	50–100 lb.
Cowpeas	40 lb.	Salsify	100 lb.
Cucumbers	120 lb.	Shallots	75 lb.
Dandelion greens	35–75 lb.	Sorrel	20–50 lb.
		Soybeans	20 lb.
Eggplants	100 lb.	Spinach	40–50 lb.
Endive	75–120 lb.	Squash, summer	100 lb.
Garden cress	15–30 lb.	Squash, winter	150 lb.
Garlic	150 bulbs	Sweet potatoes	100 lb.
Globe artichokes	150 buds	Tomatoes	100 lb.
Horseradish	60–80 roots	Turnips	50–100 lb.
Jerusalem artichokes	100 lb.	Witloof chicory	50 lb.
Kale	75–200 lb.		
Kohlrabi	75 lb.	**Tree Fruits**	**Yield per Mature Tree**
Leeks	50–100 lb.		
Lettuce, head	50 lb.	Apples, dwarf	3–5 bu.
Lettuce, leaf	50 lb.	Apples, semidwarf	4–10 bu.
Mustard greens	60–125 lb.	Apples, spur type	4–10 bu.
New Zealand spinach	50–80 lb.	Apples, standard	5–15 bu.
Okra	100 lb.	Apricots, standard	2–4 bu.
Onions	100 lb.	Cherries, sour, dwarf	2–3 pk.
Parsnips	100 lb.		

Tree Fruits	Yield per Mature Tree	Small Fruits	Yield per Plant
Cherries, sour, standard	8–12 pk.	Blackberries	2 pt.
		Blueberries	12–13 pt.
Cherries, sweet, standard	8–16 pk.	Currants	2–3 pt.
Nectarines, standard	3–5 bu.	Gooseberries	3 pt.
		Raspberries, black or purple	5 pt.
Peaches, standard	3–5 bu.		
Pears, dwarf	1–3 bu.	Raspberries, red	2 pt.
Plums, standard	3–5 bu.	Raspberries, yellow or everbearing	2 pt.
		Strawberries	2 pt.

Approximate Yield of Frozen Produce from Fresh

Vegetables	Fresh, as Purchased or Picked	Frozen
Asparagus	1 crate (12 2-lb. bunches) 1–1½ lb.	15–22 pt. 1 pt.
Beans, lima (in pods)	1 bu. (32 lb.) 2–2½ lb.	12–16 pt. 1 pt.
Beans, green, snap and wax	1 bu. (30 lb.) ⅔–1 lb.	30–45 pt. 1 pt.
Beet greens	5 lb. 1–1½ lb.	10–15 pt. 1 pt.
Beet roots	1 bu. (52 lb.) 1¼–1½ lb.	35–42 pt. 1 pt.
Broccoli	1 crate (25 lb.) 1 lb.	24 pt. 1 pt.
Brussels sprouts	4 qt. boxes 1 lb.	6 pt. 1 pt.

(continued)

Vegetables	Fresh, as Purchased or Picked	Frozen
Carrots	1 bu. (50 lb.)	32–40 pt.
	1¼–1½ lb.	1 pt.
Cauliflower	2 med. heads	3 pt.
	1⅓ lb.	1 pt.
Chard	1 bu. (12 lb.)	8–12 pt.
	1–1½ lb.	1 pt.
Collards	1 bu. (12 lb.)	8–12 pt.
	1–1½ lb.	1 pt.
Corn, sweet (in husks)	1 bu. (35 lb.)	14–17 pt.
	2–2½ lb.	1 pt.
Eggplants	1 lb.	1 pt.
Kale	1 bu. (18 lb.)	12–18 pt.
	1–1½ lb.	1 pt.
Mustard greens	1 bu. (12 lb.)	8–12 pt.
	1–1½ lb.	1 pt.
Peas (in pods)	1 bu. (30 lb.)	12–15 pt.
	2–2½ lb.	1 pt.
Peppers, sweet	⅔ lb. (3 peppers)	1 pt.
Pumpkins	3 lb.	2 pt.
Spinach	1 bu. (18 lb.)	12–18 pt.
	1–1½ lb.	1 pt.
Squash, summer	1 bu. (40 lb.)	32–40 pt.
	1–1¼ lb.	1 pt.
Squash, winter	3 lb.	2 pt.
Sweet potatoes	⅔ lb.	1 pt.

Fruits	Fresh, as Purchased or Picked	Frozen
Apples	1 bu. (48 lb.)	32–40 pt.
	1 box (44 lb.)	29–35 pt.
	1¼–1½ lb.	1 pt.

Fruits	Fresh, as Purchased or Picked	Frozen
Apricots	1 bu. (48 lb.)	60–72 pt.
	1 crate (22 lb.)	28–33 pt.
	⅔–⅘ lb.	1 pt.
Berries*	1 crate (24 qt.)	32–36 pt.
	1⅓–1½ pt.	1 pt.
Cantaloupes	1 dozen (28 lb.)	22 pt.
	1–1¼ lb.	1 pt.
Cherries, sour or sweet	1 bu. (56 lb.)	36–44 pt.
	1¼–1½ lb.	1 pt.
Cranberries	1 box (25 lb.)	50 pt.
	1 pk. (8 lb.)	16 pt.
	½ lb.	1 pt.
Currants	2 qt. (3 lb.)	4 pt.
	¾ lb.	1 pt.
Peaches	1 bu. (48 lb.)	32–48 pt.
	1 lug box (20 lb.)	13–20 pt.
	1–1½ lb.	1 pt.
Pears	1 bu. (50 lb.)	40–50 pt.
	1 western box (46 lb.)	37–46 pt.
	1–1¼ lb.	1 pt.
Plums and prunes	1 bu. (56 lb.)	38–56 pt.
	1 crate (20 lb.)	13–20 pt.
	1–1½ lb.	1 pt.
Raspberries	1 crate (24 lb.)	24 pt.
	1 pt.	1 pt.
Rhubarb	15 lb.	15–22 pt.
	⅔–1 lb.	1 pt.
Strawberries	1 crate (24 qt.)	38 pt.
	⅔ qt.	1 pt.

*Includes blackberries, blueberries, boysenberries, dewberries, elderberries, gooseberries, huckleberries, loganberries, and youngberries.

Approximate Yield of Canned Produce from Fresh

Vegetables	Fresh, as Purchased or Picked	Canned
Asparagus	1 bu. (40 lb.)	9–16 qt.
	1 crate (24 lb.)	5–10 qt.
Beans, lima (in pods)	1 bu. (32 lb.)	6–10 qt.
	1½–2½ lb.	1 pt.
Beans, snap	1 bu. (30 lb.)	12–22 qt.
	¾–1¼ lb.	1 pt.
Beet roots	1 bu. (52 lb.)	14–24 qt.
	¾–1¼ lb.	1 pt.
Cabbage	1–1½ lb.	1 pt.
Carrots	1 bu. (50 lb.)	17–20 qt.
	1–1½ lb.	1 pt.
Corn (in husks)	1 bu. (35 lb.)	6–10 qt. (kernels)
	1½–3 lb.	1 pt. (kernels)
Greens	1 bu. (18 lb.)	3–8 qt.
Okra	1 bu. (26 lb.)	17 qt.
Peas (in pods)	1 bu. (30 lb.)	5–10 qt.
	1½–2 lb.	1 pt.
Squash, summer	1 bu. (40 lb.)	10–22 qt.
	1–3 lb.	1 pt.
Squash, winter	1 bu. (11 lb.)	10–20 qt.
	¾ lb.	1 pt.
Sweet potatoes	1 bu. (50 lb.)	16–22 qt.
	1–1½ lb.	1 pt.
Tomatoes (whole)	1 bu. (53 lb.)	14–22 qt.
	1¼–1¾ lb.	1 pt.
Fruits	**Fresh, as Purchased or Picked**	**Canned**
Apples	1 bu. (48 lb.)	16–20 qt.
	2½–3 lb.	1 qt.
Apricots	1 box (22 lb.)	7–11 qt.
	2–2½ lb.	1 qt.

Fruits	Fresh, as Purchased or Picked	Canned
Berries (except strawberries)	1 crate (24 qt.) 1½–3 lb.	12–18 qt. 1 qt.
Cherries	1 bu. (56 lb.) 2–2½ lb.	22–32 qt. (unpitted) 1 qt. (unpitted)
Grapes	1 lb.	1 qt.
Peaches	1 bu. (48 lb.)	16–24 qt.
Pears	1 bu. (50 lb.)	17–25 qt.
Plums	1 bu. (56 lb.) 1½–2½ lb.	24–30 qt. 1 qt.

CHAPTER 6

Harvest, Storage, and Preparation for the Table

By the time harvest rolls around, you've expended considerable effort to assure that your garden will deliver its nutritional best.

You've been building your soil to the level where it can offer optimum amounts of vitamins and minerals to crops. You've carefully chosen varieties that offer balanced and high-quality nutrition. And you've tended those crops with loving care throughout the season. After all that, it would be a shame to lose the bulk of those stored nutrients once the crops have been harvested.

Yet, that is often what happens. Several studies have shown beyond a doubt that, despite the sometimes serious losses in vitamins and minerals that occur during the commercial growing and handling of fruits and vegetables, far greater losses are incurred after the produce reaches the kitchen. Half the job of procuring high-quality food takes place before the harvest. The other half takes place during and after harvest, right up to the time when the food disappears into your body. Both halves of this task are equally important.

Four Enemies of Nutritional Quality

In harvest, storage, and kitchen preparation, there are four major enemies of vitamins and minerals. These are heat, light, oxygen, and water.

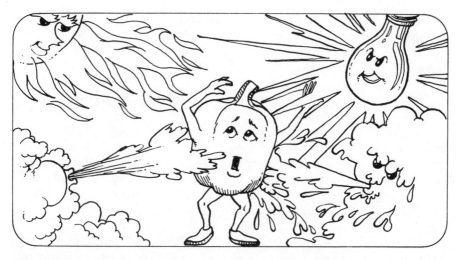

Beware of the Spoilers: *Heat, light, oxygen, and water can steal away vitamins and minerals from your harvested foods unless you take the proper precautions.*

Write these four words on a sheet of paper and attach it to your refrigerator door. *Heat, light, oxygen,* and *water.* In everything you do from the point of harvest, these will be the words to guide your actions. There are exceptions to the rules, of course, and these will be noted. But, in general, the less your garden products are subjected to heat, light, oxygen, and water, the better they'll be able to retain their original stores of vitamins and minerals.

The Perfect Harvest Point

When is a tomato absolutely ripe? When does a melon contain the optimum amount of vitamin A? When should an eggplant be cut from the plant for top flavor and vitamin content? When is a snow pea ready to leave the vine?

Long-time gardeners have learned through experience when each crop is at its peak of flavor and texture: the tomato when it is dead ripe and before its skin begins to take on a wrinkled look; the melon when it can be separated easily from the vine with gentle thumb pressure; the eggplant when it seems fairly bursting within itself and before the black skin has begun to lose its sheen; the snow pea just as the first bumps of the seeds show through the pods. (For guidelines on how to judge the perfect harvest point for other vegetables, fruits, and nuts, see chapter 7.)

Fortunately, nature has provided us with crops that usually reach their peak of nutritional goodness just as they reach their most attractive and tasteful stage. This is a gift that stood our primitive forebears in good stead, since they knew much more about what looked and tasted good than about the virtues of ascorbic acid and provitamin A. Again, however, there are exceptions to the rule. And if you are to plan your harvest for peak nutritional value, it is the exceptions which you must remember and heed.

Sunshine Builds Vitamin C

Light is the enemy of vitamins after crops have been harvested. But before they are harvested, while they are still part of a living and growing plant, light is a valuable ally in building stores of vitamin C.

Ascorbic acid, after all, is a sugar derivative. The sugars in a plant are manufactured during photosynthesis, and photosynthesis requires light. The more light, therefore, the more sugar—and the more vitamin C— is manufactured.

Scientists have found that a food crop will lose vitamin C in darkness or in reduced light and will regain vitamin C when exposed again to strong light. Beans lose 20 percent of their vitamin C when placed in total darkness for only 24 hours. But they will regain what they've lost when exposed again to light. Peppers have less vitamin C during the night than they do during the day. Kale was found to lose some vitamin C late in the season, when the days were growing shorter. Peas planted close together contained less ascorbic acid than those spaced farther apart, a result of the pods being shaded. Tomatoes grown continuously in the sun had 40 percent more vitamin C than those grown in the shade. And tomatoes ripened in the shade of their own leaves had less vitamin C than those ripened in full sun. All of these findings were reported by researchers G. Fred Somers and Kenneth C. Beeson of the U.S. Plant, Soil and Nutrition Laboratory in Ithaca, New York.[1]

The lesson to be learned in harvesting is to pick crops after they have been exposed to as much sunlight as possible. A cloudy day following several other cloudy days is not the best time to harvest crops for high vitamin C content. If possible, wait for a day of sunshine, and then harvest the crop in the afternoon, while the sun is still fairly high in the sky. Remember that vitamin C can be built up or reduced in a matter of hours—not only days—and that proper timing may result in a bonus of 20 percent or more vitamin C from every crop you pick. (You should also be aware that the highest levels of ascorbic acid are found on the outer surfaces of plants, where photosynthesis takes place.)

Generally, ascorbic acid level increases as the food portions of crops grow to maturity, then begins to fall. This has been shown to be true in the cases of tomatoes, peppers, snap beans, and peas and presumably is true for other vegetables and fruits. The ascorbic acid content of white potatoes and beets, however, remains constant during their growth. There's no need to worry about shortchanging nutrient benefits when you harvest immature beets and new potatoes for use during the growing season. Strawberries have very little vitamin C before they develop their red color, then it increases rapidly and remains constant until full maturity, when the vitamin C level begins to fall back. The key here is to harvest strawberries anytime they are red, but before they approach overripeness, for high vitamin C value.

Catching Nutrient Levels at Their Peak

The B vitamins are generally found in highest amounts in actively growing shoots of plants and in seed embryos. Mature tissues hold relatively little of the B vitamins. In vegetables, B vitamin levels don't seem to change significantly during the maturation process. Most important here are the kinds of crops you grow, not the time of harvest.

Provitamin A, or carotene, increases in carrots, peppers, tomatoes, and yellow corn during maturation, but sweet potatoes are believed to hold a consistent level during the growing season. The beautiful thing about provitamin A is that you can actually see the orange-colored carotene in the plant and can therefore judge for yourself how rich in vitamin A that food is. A Caro-Red tomato, which has about ten times the carotene content of a standard red tomato, for instance, is bright orange in color precisely because of its high carotene content. Carrots that are deep orange in color are richer in vitamin A than pale orange-yellow carrots. The Imperator carrot, which is exceptionally high in carotene, was bred for its rich color, which was judged to have supermarket appeal—not for its high vitamin content, which was merely a happy concurrence. As tomatoes and peppers change from green to red, you should recognize that their green chlorophyll is being replaced by orange carotene. Muskmelons, peaches, and apricots have peak vitamin A values when their flesh is at its deepest shade of orange. For all these crops, let your eyes be the judge of vitamin A value, and harvest accordingly.

The level of all minerals increases as food crops reach maturity, but this is because at maturity crops tend to have less water and a higher ash content, which is the mineral matter. But the difference in the mineral amounts between an almost-ripe and a dead-ripe vegetable is not significant. In essence, mineral content is not greatly affected by the time of harvest.

Protein levels, in general, increase with the advancing maturity of the crop. At the same time, the amino acid profile remains constant. For maximum protein content, then, it's best to wait until crops are at full maturity. And since many of the garden crops you depend on for protein are seeds and nuts, which are often left to dry on the plant or tree, full maturity poses no problem. Amaranth, broccoli, peas, and potatoes, which are also good protein sources, should be harvested as needed when they reach good table quality. Any slight losses in protein incurred when you harvest these crops at an immature stage will not be significant in your total food plan.

When the Fruit Leaves the Vine

As soon as the fruit leaves the vine, quality begins to deteriorate. It's at this time that the four enemies of vitamins and minerals come into play: heat, light, oxygen, and water.

Unless you spread a picnic blanket down in the middle of the garden and eat your dinner directly from the plants around you, your garden foods are going to lose some nutritional quality between the time of harvest and the time of eating. It is inevitable. But it's your job to organize the harvest so that the loss in quality is as slight as possible.

When the fruit leaves the vine, the fruit does not die. It continues to respire. Chemical changes take place. Enzyme activity continues. The fruit continues to ripen. It is still a living thing, but now it is a living entity unto itself, cut off from the vital support of the mother plant. Now the harvested fruit can be affected much more easily by environmental conditions, namely heat, light, oxygen, and water.

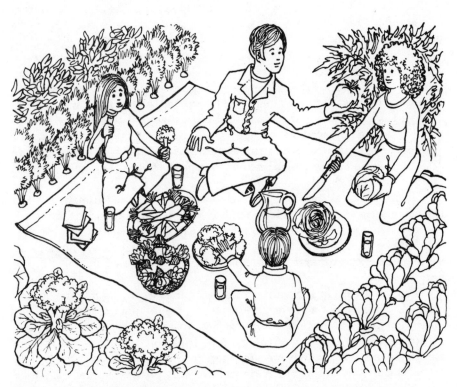

Dinnertime in the Garden: *The only way your homegrown food won't lose nutrients between harvest and mealtime is if you eat it right in the garden. Short of dining al fresco, there are steps you can take to hold nutrient losses to a minimum.*

The most vulnerable of all nutritional elements at this time is vitamin C. All plants contain oxidase systems which can oxidize ascorbic acid, destroying it or reducing its quality. Unfavorable environmental conditions, including heat and cold, exposure to air (with resultant wilting), and physical damage act to induce stress conditions in the plant tissues. And this tissue stress accelerates the oxidation of vitamin C. (On the other hand, light is not an enemy of vitamin C at this stage—quite the opposite, as we soon shall see.)

There are gardeners who, before going out to harvest sweet corn, start the pot boiling in the kitchen. They then race back to the kitchen with the corn, husk it quickly, and drop it into the steam basket within minutes. They do this because they know that immediately after leaving the mother plant, the kernels of corn begin to change their sugar to starch, thus lowering quality of taste and texture.

Follow this example and treat all your harvesting as these gardeners treat corn. You don't necessarily have to race back to a boiling pot with all your garden vegetables, but the sooner you can get them into the kitchen and use them, the more vitamins and minerals, as well as quality of taste and texture, you will preserve.

Wilting—the result of exposure to heat and oxygen—is devastating to vitamin C, especially in leafy crops which have a very high surface area in relationship to their mass. Two researchers conducted studies on kale and reported their findings in volume 7 of the *Journal of Agricultural Food Chemistry*. Left in a 70°F room for two days, kale will lose 89 percent of its ascorbic acid. Of course, you would never leave a bunch of kale on the kitchen counter for two days, but remember that the destruction of vitamin C begins as soon as the leaves are separated from the root system and that it proceeds apace from that point on. If you've ever left just-harvested leafy crops to lie in the garden row in the hot sun for an hour while you harvested other vegetables, you were actually helping to promote rampant vitamin loss.

The main culprit here is heat. If the same kale were to be kept at a temperature of 32°F, all other factors being equal, the loss of vitamin C would be only 5 percent. A good scheme when harvesting kale, endive, collards, lettuce, and other leafy crops is to fill a washtub with cold water from the garden hose and drop the leaves into the water as they are harvested. Then, when the job is finished, remove the leaves from the water, shake off the excess, and carry them home in a paper bag. There will be some slight vitamin C loss from contact with the water, but nothing compared to the oxidation caused by exposure to the afternoon sun and air. This chilling-in-the-field process is a good one for many other crops with the exception of sweet potatoes, okra, cucumbers, snap beans, peppers, eggplants, and tomatoes. All of these vegetables are chill susceptible and stand to lose more ascorbic acid from the shock of being chilled than from any short-term wilting. Cabbage, squash, and root crops are fairly well

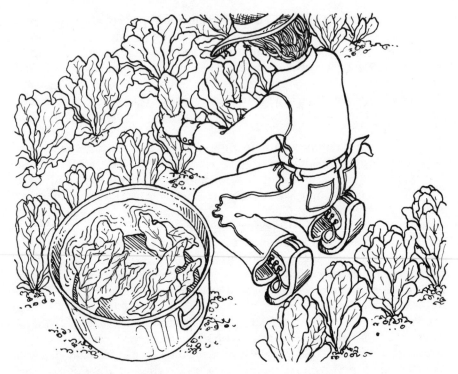

Give Leafy Greens a Chill: *Plunging harvested leafy greens immediately into a tub of cold water is the best way to safeguard their vitamin C content.*

protected from wilting by their very structure and do not need chilling in the field.

When you reach home with the harvested vegetables and fruits, prepare them for the table or for storage as quickly as possible. Never harvest several bushels of crops that you hope to can or freeze sometime during the following several days, particularly if the weather is warm. Even if your garden is a good distance from your home, it will be worth your while to make more trips and put up smaller batches of better-quality foods. If you have a small garden at home and a larger one at a distance, consider raising wilt-vulnerable leafy crops at home and the rest of the crops in the main garden for maximum vitamin C retention.

While vegetables are awaiting your attention in the kitchen, be sure to refrigerate them immediately, except for the chill-susceptible vegetables mentioned earlier. Keep beans and peas in the pods, and don't trim away any outer leaves from vegetables such as endive and cabbage before refrigerating if you can avoid it. Follow all these steps and you will offset the effects of the four major enemies of vitamins and minerals.

Storing Foods for Quality

The principles applied to harvesting crops are carried through in preparing them for canning, freezing, and drying and for short-term storage in the kitchen, as well.

For short-term storage, depend on your refrigerator for best nutrient retention. Cold temperatures slow down respiration, enzyme activity, and the actions of microorganisms. By slowing down these natural processes you help retain vitamins and minerals in crops. In short-term storage, vitamin C is again the most vulnerable nutrient. The loss of vitamin C, in fact, is in almost direct proportion to the increase in temperature.

Even in the refrigerator, vitamin C losses are significant. One study showed that, at refrigerator temperatures between 40° and 50°F, green beans lost 10 percent of their ascorbic acid in 24 hours. Broccoli lost 10 to 30 percent, chard 30 percent, and spinach 19 percent.[2] On the other hand, sweet corn lost none of its vitamin C when refrigerated in the husk nor did carrots when they were refrigerated for long periods. Corn and carrots, however, contain relatively little vitamin C in any case.

There is not much information available on the stability of the B vitamins in storage. We do know that there is very little loss of thiamine and riboflavin, even when vegetables are exposed to room temperatures for several days. Folic acid, on the other hand, is easily destroyed. When held at room temperature for three days, endive lost 71 percent of its folic acid, spinach lost 41 percent, asparagus 73 percent, and green beans 56 percent.[3]

Vitamin A is not easily lost in carrots, sweet potatoes, and squash during storage. However, leafy vegetables lose vitamin A quickly when exposed to wilting conditions.

Both washing and trimming of vegetables and fruits leads to very quick loss of vitamin C as well as some other nutrients. For this reason, you should never wash, trim, or cut them in any way until it's actually time to prepare them for table use or long-term storage. Specifically, this means you should store corn in the husk; leave beans and peas in the pods; keep cabbage without removing any more of its outer leaves than necessary to fit the head into the refrigerator; hold melons and squash whole and uncut; and store strawberries with their caps and stems attached.

Cutting, chopping, and mincing vegetables exposes them quickly to air and leads to very rapid vitamin and mineral depletion. To avoid this nutrient loss, vegetables should not be cut for freezing, canning, or table use until the very last minute. If coleslaw is on the menu for tonight, prepare other foods ahead of time—but don't mince or shred the cabbage until just before dinner. When preparing snap beans, don't French cut them, since this exposes the tender inner part of the pods to oxygen. For salads, quarter the tomatoes instead of slicing them thinly, for best nutrient retention. Cook broccoli and cauliflower whole without breaking them up

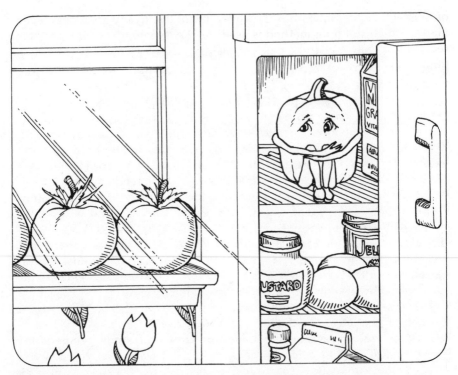

To Each Its Own: *If you won't be using a garden-fresh pepper for a while, store it in the refrigerator, not out on the counter. Fewer nutrients will be lost through chilling than would be lost through wilting. When you bring tomatoes that are not quite ripe into the kitchen, let them ripen at room temperature on a sunny windowsill. You'll boost their vitamin C content this way.*

into florets first. In all your food preparations, insofar as possible, try to protect the surface area of fruits and vegetables from exposure to air.

As you recall from the earlier discussion of chilling harvested crops in the garden, it's best not to subject chill-susceptible vegetables to cold temperatures. In general, these are the vegetables of tropical origin, known as the warm-weather crops: okra, cucumbers, snap beans, peppers, eggplants, and tomatoes. Depending on the room temperature and the length of time the vegetables are to be exposed, however, it may be better to refrigerate cucumbers, snap beans, and peppers. When it comes to a choice between wilting and chilling, sometimes it is better to chill.

In the case of tomatoes, the facts are now well known. They should be ripened on a sunny windowsill at room temperature. A tomato ripened in this way will contain 50 percent more vitamin C than one ripened at similar temperatures in the dark.[4] Gardeners who were taught to ripen tomatoes by wrapping them in newspaper and storing them on a basement shelf will discontinue the practice if they care about the nutritional quality of their tomatoes. (Vitamin A, however, is not lost to any great degree, no matter which ripening method is used. As the tomato turns from green to red, both vitamins A and C tend to increase to some extent, whether the tomato is in the sun or not.)

Freezing Fruits and Vegetables

Except for a few fruits and vegetables better suited to the root cellar, freezing is the best way to preserve vitamins and minerals. When plant tissues are brought down to the zero point and oxygen is completely screened off, all biological activity comes to a virtual halt, and the plant rests in a state of suspended activity. Even at 0°F, however, there are some internal changes, which is why foods cannot be kept frozen indefinitely and still retain their quality. The best practice is to freeze only enough of any crop to last for one year. The vitamins most vulnerable to losses while frozen are vitamin C, riboflavin, pantothenic acid (one of the B vitamins), and in some cases vitamin A.

Freezer temperature is of critical importance. In one experiment, peas stored for one year at 0°F lost 20 percent of their vitamin C. Stored at 10°F, the peas lost 83 percent of vitamin C in one year. At 20°F, they lost 83 percent in only two months. And at 30°F—still freezing temperature— they lost 83 percent in *two weeks*.[5]

Experiments with other fruits and vegetables show similar results, although some hold vitamin C more efficiently than others. In every case, losses were relatively small at 0°F but increased quickly at temperatures above 10°F.

This sensitivity of food to temperatures even well within the freezing range is reason enough for you to check your freezing unit very carefully. Many older freezers are very inefficient, requiring significant amounts of energy to keep foods frozen—and then at temperatures well above the desired zero-or-below mark. Freezing units of refrigerators are notoriously unreliable, particularly in older models, whose seals might have begun to deteriorate. Check your own freezer each year, placing reliable outdoor thermometers in several places within the unit, leaving them there overnight before checking temperatures. If your freezer registers much above 0°F, it might be time to consider investing in a new energy-efficient model, one that is guaranteed to hold foods at subzero temperatures. At the very least, you should repair faulty seals so your freezer can work as efficiently as possible.

Blanching foods (exposing them to intense heat for a short period) before freezing can result in a loss of up to 60 percent of water-soluble vitamins and minerals. Nevertheless, blanching is absolutely necessary if fruits and vegetables are to retain their quality in the frozen state. Anyone who has tried to freeze foods without blanching them first knows that most soon become rubbery and tasteless, losing all of their fresh character.

Unblanched frozen foods also lose vitamins and minerals at an alarming rate so that, after only a few weeks, they are more depleted than their blanched counterparts. (Some exceptions are peppers, chives, and many herbs, which may be frozen without blanching.)

The main benefit of blanching is that it inactivates enzymes and kills bacteria that cause losses in quality. Freezing slows down these enzymes but cannot inactivate them to the degree necessary for long-term storage, as exposure to high temperatures can. In the blanching process, however, you must accept an inevitable loss of vitamins and minerals because of the exposure of the foods to heat, oxygen, and water.

You can lessen the degree of vitamin and mineral loss by steam blanching foods. In steam blanching, nutrient loss due to leaching is held to a minimum because the foods do not come into direct contact with the boiling water. Oxidation losses are small also, because the lid on the pot traps air inside. Of course, you should realize that there will be nutrients lost due to heat exposure, especially since steam-blanched vegetables are exposed to heat longer than water-blanched ones.

Steam blanching is not difficult. You can use a pressure cooker or a large kettle or pot. You need a wire basket or colander which fits into the pot to hold the vegetables above the boiling water. After you've washed and trimmed the vegetables, place them in the basket in a layer no more than 2 inches deep. Keep at least 2 inches of water boiling rapidly to generate a maximum amount of steam, and keep the pot covered while the vegetables are steaming.

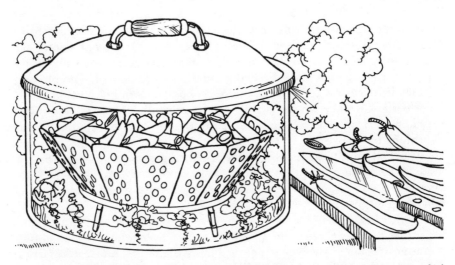

Steam Blanching: *If you'll be freezing some of the harvest, try steam blanching instead of the usual water blanching. Nutrient loss will be kept to a minimum since the food doesn't come in contact with the boiling water.*

Freezing — Quick, Quick, Quick

These pointers will help you concentrate on the steps in the freezing process that will result in the greatest conservation of nutrients. The secrets to nutrition-wise freezing are nothing more than *organization* and *quickness*.

• Be sure you have all your tools and utensils ready beforehand. While you are searching for your old colander or running to the neighbor's to borrow some ice, oxidation of vitamin C continues.

• Don't bring home more produce than you can freeze in an afternoon. The shortest time between the vine and the freezer results in foods of highest nutritional quality.

• Wash vegetables and fruits quickly and with a minimum amount of water. Never soak them in water.

• Keep produce in the refrigerator until it's time to prepare it for freezing.

• Blanch thoroughly, but don't overblanch.

• Organize the procedure so that foods are washed, trimmed, blanched, cooled, and packed into containers with as little delay as possible between steps. A two- or three-person team works best.

• Freeze the foods as quickly as possible. When placing containers in the freezing unit, leave plenty of room for air to circulate around each container. Investigate quick freezing foods on cookie sheets before they are packed into containers; this is especially useful with blueberries and strawberries.

Each piece of food should be heated through, and the idea is to do it as quickly as possible, since time is an important factor in vitamin and mineral loss, no matter what the cause. Food scientists found that vegetables retained 88 to 100 percent of their vitamin C when steam blanched, 64 to 95 percent in short-term water blanching, but as little as 6 percent when foods were water blanched in a large amount of water for an extended period.[6] Other studies have shown that blanching also removes B vitamins and minerals in varying amounts and that steam blanching conserves all of these nutrients most effectively. (Tests have shown also that microwave blanching results in vitamin and mineral retention equal to, but not better than, steam blanching. But since there are safety questions regarding microwave ovens, we cannot recommend the practice here.)

After foods have been blanched, they must be cooled as quickly as possible in order to avoid further nutrient losses. The time-honored practice of dumping fruits and vegetables into a tub of ice water is a major destroyer of water-soluble vitamins and minerals. Nutrients leach out into the ice water at an especially rapid rate when the foods are hot and have a high amount of surface area (due to trimming and cutting). A better idea is to fill one pan—perhaps a large baking pan—with water and ice and float a smaller but similarly shaped pan on top of it. Spread out the blanched food in the top pan and cover it immediately with plastic bags full of ice cubes.

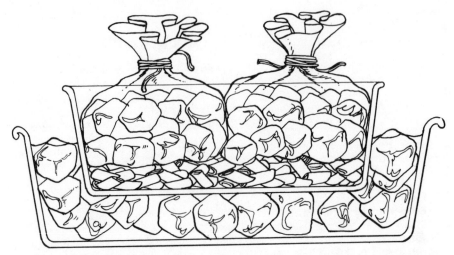

Cooling Blanched Foods: *Don't dump just-blanched foods directly into a tub of water to cool them quickly. Protect their nutrient content by sandwiching them between two chilly layers of cold water and ice cubes. Because the food doesn't come in direct contact with the water and ice, no nutrients are leached away.*

Iced on both top and bottom, the food will cool quickly with no further exposure to water and no further leaching. (For this procedure, you'll probably want to begin storing up ice cubes during the preceding week.)

Canning—Sealing in Goodness

Vegetables and fruits prepared for canning lose more vitamins and minerals than those prepared for freezing because of the longer exposure to heat in the sterilization process. In one experiment, peas lost 5 percent of their vitamin C content when frozen but 16.7 percent when canned. Nevertheless, once foods are actually sealed in the jars, they are able to hold a very high percentage of their nutrients when stored at ordinary room temperatures. The 1959 United States Department of Agriculture *Handbook of Agriculture* reported that canned fruits and vegetables lose very little vitamin C when stored at 65°F, no more than 10 percent after a full year. When stored at 80°F, however, vitamin C loss increased to 25 percent. Canning actually seals in nutritional goodness quite well if the cans are kept in a cool, dark place. In some cases, canning is superior to freezing in this respect.

In the canning process, exposure to temperatures of boiling or above kill all pathogenic and spoilage organisms that may be present in the food. Storage in sterilized, airtight jars keeps the food well protected after that. High-acid foods such as fruits, pickled vegetables, and tomatoes are susceptible only to heat-sensitive organisms. Low-acid foods (a category which includes most other vegetables), however, are susceptible also to some potentially harmful organisms that cannot be killed by the 212°F temperature of ordinary boiling. The most feared of these organisms is *Clostridium botulinum*, which forms a dangerous toxin that causes botulism. Because of this danger, low-acid foods should be processed in a pressure canner which can produce the 240°F temperature needed to kill all traces of *C. botulinum*. Although the higher-than-boiling temperatures of the pressure canner are hard on heat-sensitive vitamins, including folic acid, thiamine, and vitamin A, the process is necessary in home canning.

Vitamin and mineral losses can be held to a minimum by processing the foods in the shortest time possible. University of Minnesota food scientists Edmund A. Zottola and Isabel D. Wolf recommend pressure canning at 15 pounds of pressure to the square inch rather than the 10 pounds commonly recommended. By reducing the time foods need for processing, losses of nutrients are also reduced. This method is recom-

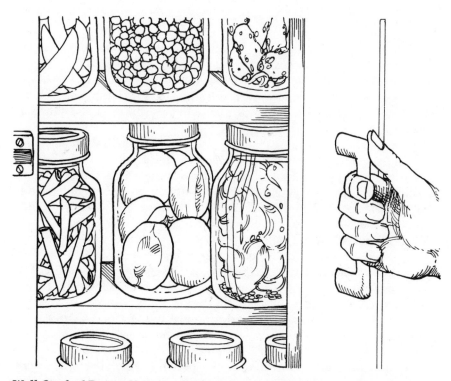

Well-Stocked Pantry: *How you treat foods once they're processed can affect their nutrient content. Store canning jars in a cool, dark place to keep heat and light from stealing nutrients.*

mended for both high- and low-acid foods and vegetables and is safe to use in the kitchen (although, of course, your pressure canner must be in good working order).

When you can foods, attempt to limit the air space at the top of the jar to the lowest permissible level. Even the slight amount of oxygen contained in the air space will act to oxidize ascorbic acid during storage. Then, be sure to store the jars in a cool and dark place. Heat and light definitely are enemies at this stage.

During storage, fruits and vegetables packed in sterilized water "lose" great amounts of the water-soluble vitamins and minerals. These nutrients have nowhere to go, of course, except to the water in the jar. After just a few weeks in storage, the vitamin C in a jar of peas will be half in the water and half in the peas themselves. Be sure to cook vegetables in the water they were stored in, and then try to use that water in soup stocks or in other recipes.

Organization and quickness are just as important when you're canning as when you're freezing. The less time your foods are exposed to heat, light, oxygen, and water, the more nutrients they will retain.

Drying Foods

Food dehydration has some definite advantages. It's an easy preservation method to carry out, and the dried foods can be stored easily and economically in very little space. Dried foods are a boon to backpackers, and some specialty foods such as fruit leathers may be created only in this way. Dried fruits are a wholesome and delicious snack, a good substitute for candy.

As with any method of food preservation, dehydration has some drawbacks, nutritionally speaking. Because the drying process requires long exposure to air and heat, various nutrients, such as vitamin C, some of the B complex, and provitamin A are lost. Sulfur, used to prevent browning and ascorbic acid loss in dried fruits, also destroys thiamine. In addition, foods to be dried are usually blanched and sliced thin (so they will dry quickly), creating further nutrient loss.

Vitamin A losses in dried foods may be major. Anyone who has dried carrots has noticed that, during the process, the yellow-orange color of the roots fades quickly away. This is, in fact, the very carotene which provides provitamin A being carried away with the moisture. Spinach, another rich provider of A, loses almost all of it during the drying process. Dried sweet peppers stored for 19 months were shown to lose 80 percent of their vitamin A. Apricots lose 66 to 82 percent.[7]

Among the B vitamins, thiamine is especially vulnerable to air drying. (If a food is first treated with sulfur, then air dried, most of the thiamine will be gone before it is even put away for storage.) Other B vitamins are somewhat less vulnerable. Experimenters reported losses of less than 10 percent of riboflavin, niacin, and pantothenic acid in various air-dried vegetables after blanching.[8]

Vitamin C, the most unstable nutrient and also the one we depend most on fruits and vegetables for, is attacked at every stage of the drying process. This loss can be largely compensated for if fruits are pretreated with vitamin C (dipped in a solution of 2,000 milligrams powdered ascorbic acid to 1 quart water), but this is tantamount to fortifying your own garden foods, which should not be necessary in a home food system. It also does not replace rutin, a valuable ascorbic acid companion.

Vitamins Underground

Root cellaring and other underground storage methods are excellent ways to preserve vitamins and minerals in those crops suited to such storage. Potatoes and other root crops are the most common candidates, but cabbage, kohlrabi, squash, and pumpkins are also suited to root cellaring, as are some apples and pears.

The beauty of root cellaring is that the process requires no trimming, cutting, mincing, blanching, boiling, pressure cooking, or any of the other procedures that devastate vitamins and minerals. The only nutrients lost will be through the skins of the vegetables and fruits due to slow exposure to surrounding air and through internal biological changes.

This book won't go into a full discussion of root cellaring, since the information is readily available elsewhere. The chart on Energy-Saving Storage of Vegetables and Fruits will give you some guidelines to follow, and the Recommended Reading list at the back of the book can steer you toward some helpful books. In general, cooler temperatures enable stored crops to retain a greater percentage of their vitamins and minerals. An environment just above freezing is usually recommended, with a relative humidity level of 70 to 90 percent.

A major exception to the temperature rule is found in the case of potato storage. Although the potato is not the richest of garden crops in vitamin and mineral content, it is the greatest contributor to our diets of many nutrients, just because we happen to eat so many potatoes. It will pay rich nutritional dividends, then, to offer just the right storage conditions for the autumn potato harvest.

A temperature between 34° and 41°F has traditionally been recommended for potatoes since this range retards sprouting. Scientific investigation, however, has found that potatoes retain much more vitamin C when stored at higher temperatures. Those stored at 40°F lost as much ascorbic acid in two months as those stored at 50° or 60°F lost in five months.[9] One particular study showed that white potatoes stored for six months in a cool, damp cellar (37° to 40°F) lost 30 to 50 percent of ascorbic acid, while those stored for the same period in a warm, dry cellar (55° to 60°F) showed a loss between 0 and 20 percent.[10]

(continued on page 130)

Energy-Saving Storage of Vegetables and Fruits

Produce	Place to Store*	Storage Period	Temperature**	Humidity
Vegetables				
Dry beans and peas	Any cool, dry place	As long as desired	Cool	Dry
Late cabbage	Outdoor pit or trench; indoor storage cellar	Through late fall and winter	Cool	Moderately moist
Cauliflower and broccoli	Any cold place	2–3 weeks	32°F	Moderately moist
Late celery	Outdoor pit or trench; roots in slightly moist soil or sand in cellar	Through late fall and winter	Cool	Moist
Endive	Roots in soil in cellar	2–3 months	Cool	Moist
Onions	Any cool, dry place	Through fall and winter	Cool	Dry
Parsnips	Mulched in garden row; indoor storage cellar	Through fall and winter	Cold; freezing in soil does not injure roots	Moist
Potatoes	Outdoor pit; indoor storage cellar	Through fall and winter	See text	Dry to moderately moist

*Always avoid contact with free water that may condense and drip from ceilings.

**Cool indicates a temperature anywhere between 32° and 40°F; avoid freezing.

Produce	Place to Store*	Storage Period	Temperature**	Humidity
Pumpkins and squash	Moderately dry indoor storage cellar or basement	Through late fall and winter	50°–60°F	Moderately dry
Various root crops	Outdoor pit; indoor storage cellar	Through fall and winter	Cool	Moist
Sweet potatoes	Moderately dry indoor storage cellar or basement	Through fall and winter	55°–60°F	Moderately dry
Tomatoes (mature green)	Moderately dry indoor storage cellar or basement	4–6 weeks	55°–60°F	Moderately dry
Fruits				
Apples	Outdoor pit; indoor storage cellar or basement	Through fall and winter	Cool	Moderately moist
Grapes	Indoor storage cellar or basement	1–2 months	Cool	Moderately moist
Peaches	Indoor storage cellar or basement	2–4 weeks	31°–32°F	Moderately moist

(continued)

Energy-Saving Storage—*continued*

Produce	Place to Store*	Storage Period	Temperature**	Humidity
Fruits—continued				
Pears	Indoor storage cellar	Depends on variety; anywhere from 8 weeks to several months	Cool	Moderately moist
Plums	Indoor storage cellar or basement	4–6 weeks	Cool	Moderately moist

Other studies show that potatoes in storage hold B vitamins very efficiently. In fact, some members of the B complex, particularly vitamin B_6, increase with storage. Part of the increase can no doubt be attributed to some loss of water within the potato (thus giving higher readings of all solids), but also responsible are continuing enzyme activities within the living root. Potatoes also show a marked increase in vitamin C after they begin to sprout, again the result of enzyme activity.

The problem for home gardeners, then, is how to store potatoes at temperatures high enough to preserve vitamin C efficiently yet low enough to prevent sprouting. A good plan might be to store them for the long term under cool conditions, then bring them into a warmer room for several weeks before you intend to use them in the kitchen. In this way, sprouting will be avoided, and the time spent in the warmer air will promote the desired increase in ascorbic acid.

Preparing Foods for the Table

Collards are an excellent source of calcium, vitamin A, the B complex, and vitamin C—a nutritional powerhouse, in other words. But if you decide to "boil up a mess of greens," stewing the collards for an hour or two, the resulting dish will be reduced from a powerhouse to a nutritional blackout. Most of the vitamins and minerals that were not destroyed by the long exposure to heat will have leached into the cooking water. In this case, you would be better off to throw away the collards and drink the water. At least you would have a nutritious, low-calorie drink.

Remember the enemies heat, light, oxygen, and water? The same principles discussed earlier in this chapter apply equally to the preparation of foods for the table. Here, too, *time* is a critical factor. The more quickly fresh fruits and vegetables go from their natural state to the dinner table, the more nutritional quality they will retain. And the more quickly foods are cooked, the more nutritious they will be. Let's start from the logical point—bringing food into the kitchen—and go from there through all the various steps that lead from the kitchen to the dinner table.

As mentioned in an earlier section, When the Fruit Leaves the Vine, most fruits and vegetables should be refrigerated as soon as they reach the kitchen to slow down their enzymatic activities and prevent rapid oxidation, especially of vitamin C. For short-term storage, plastic or paper bags will help stop oxygen contact. A good vegetable crisper is a blessing. Lacking one, pick up some inexpensive plastic storage bins that have airtight lids.

Fruits and vegetables should be washed before they are trimmed or cut for the cooking pot. In washing all your organically grown fruits and

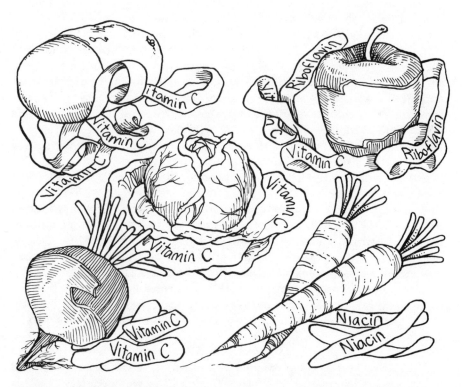

Go Easy with the Paring Knife: *The less you trim and peel your fruits and vegetables, the more vitamins and minerals they will retain. Many nutrients are found in higher concentrations in the outer leaves and surface layers.*

vegetables, strive for a least-is-best policy. Wash them quickly and use as little water as possible. Don't scrub potatoes under running water, but wipe them with a soft cloth, then rinse very quickly. Gourmet cooks tell you to wash mushrooms using a soft damp cloth to preserve their delicate flavor. Their nutritional goodness will be preserved in this way, also. However, if you've purchased produce that might contain pesticide residues, turn to a safe-is-best policy and scrub it thoroughly. And if fruits or vegetables are paraffin coated, be sure to peel them before using.

Trimming is a major source of vitamin and mineral loss, particularly since many nutrients are found in a far higher concentration in the outer leaves of vegetables and in the surface layers of roots and fruits. When your mother, in an attempt to get you to eat your potato skins, told you that all the vitamins were there, she was close to the truth. By peeling the skin from a potato, you lose from 12 to 35 percent of the ascorbic acid.[11] The outer leaves of lettuce and cabbage are higher in vitamin C than the paler inner leaves. Don't trim and toss them away as a matter of course. By peeling and slicing beets, you lose 50 percent of the vitamin C.[12] Vitamin C levels are three to ten times higher in the skin of an apple than in the inner flesh. Niacin and riboflavin are also richer in the apple's peel. In carrots, niacin in particular is concentrated in the surface tissues. If you wash a carrot well, there's no need to peel it at all. Broccoli leaves have about 40 times as much vitamin A value as the stalks and several times as much as the coveted flower heads. Don't automatically cut away and discard the small and tender leaves nestling around the stalk; they have a good flavor and they greatly enhance the total nutritional package. In general, attempt to retain as much of the outer portions of crops as you possibly can. This might require quite a change in attitude, since most of us were taught to peel virtually everything before eating it, but the nutritional rewards will be well worth the effort of this minor attitudinal change.

After fruits and vegetables are washed and trimmed, they are often sliced, chopped, diced, minced, and run through blenders or food processors, and otherwise broken down into varying-size pieces. All these operations rupture cells in plant tissues and expose the plant's moisture to oxygen, resulting in rapid vitamin and mineral depletion. Of course, vegetables cut into smaller pieces require less cooking time and there is less vitamin loss by thermal destruction, so there is a trade-off. But in general, don't cut up foods any more than you must. Particularly if they are to be eaten raw, in salads or perhaps with a dip, they should be cut into large pieces—tomatoes quartered rather than sliced, radishes served whole, lettuce torn into large pieces. Let the salad eater do the cutting in the bowl, and the nutritional package will be stronger.

Standing time in the kitchen is critical. The loss after fruits and vegetables are trimmed and cut is due to air and/or water contact. Potatoes peeled and stored in the refrigerator for five hours lose 12 percent of their thiamine, and sweet potatoes lose 21 percent. A refrigerated cantaloupe holds its nutritional value very well—but if it is sliced, bagged, and refrigerated for 24 hours, it loses 35 percent of its vitamin C.[13] In general, the vitamins most susceptible to loss in standing time are ascorbic acid, thiamine, and riboflavin, although other vitamins, and minerals, too, are lost by this exposure to air and/or water. Meats, cheeses, and grain products are far less susceptible to nutritional deterioration than are fruits and vegetables. In your food preparation plan, organize your activities to recognize this fact. Prepare ahead of time those foods that are more nutritionally stable, and make up the salad and steam the vegetable just before you call the family to dinner.

Cooking Quickly Means Eating Well

Although vitamins and minerals are inevitably lost in cooking, the total average loss here is not as great as it is in all the steps undertaken in the kitchen *before* the actual cooking process. In cooking, as in preparation, you can adopt practices to hold vitamin and mineral losses to a minimum. And again, the key is—quick, quick, quick. The quicker foods are cooked, the fewer nutrients are lost.

Before you decide which cooking methods to use, consider cooking less. Since all fruits are delicious when eaten raw, there is really very little excuse to subject them to cooking at all. Consider, first, simply putting a household ban on the cooking of fruits. An occasional hot apple pie might be a permissible treat, but there are many recipes for fruit pies that don't require cooking that can win your heart, as well.

In addition, you can eat more vegetables in their raw state. Consider increasing your consumption of salads, using more vegetables than the traditional lettuce, tomatoes, cucumbers, onions, radishes, and peppers. Use cauliflower, broccoli, spinach, tender green beans, young amaranth leaves, tender dandelions, kohlrabi, parsnips, and nearly any other fresh garden vegetables. Try cold vegetable soups, and if you have a juicer, take advantage of hearty vegetable juice concoctions. You may hesitate to run raw vegetables through a juicer or food processor, recalling the point that was made earlier that destroying plant cells leads to vitamin and mineral losses by oxygen exposure. But remember, too, that nutrient loss begins to take place *immediately after* the food is processed. It is not the actual processing that destroys vitamins and minerals, but the exposure to air and light afterward. If you eat or drink the foods immediately after processing, nutrient loss will be minimal—certainly less than it would be after cooking.

When you cook vegetables, the highest percentage of nutrients will be preserved if you cook them as quickly as possible in as little water as possible. Long-term boiling in generous amounts of water is death to many vitamins and minerals. But pressure cooking, steaming, and quick frying (French or Oriental style) are all very good methods.

If you cook vegetables in water, use just the bare minimum of water. One-half cup should be sufficient for a four-person serving of any vegetable. Get the water boiling rapidly, then add the vegetable, fresh or frozen, put a lid on the pot, and turn the heat down low. Remember that after the water is boiling, foods won't cook any more quickly with high heat than with low heat since a temperature of 212°F will be maintained in either case. Learn to judge the amount of cooking water so that there is virtually none left in the pot after the vegetable is ready for the table.

A better idea is to cook without placing the vegetable directly in water. Steaming is a method growing in popularity, and for good reason. Here, you place the vegetable on a rack above a few inches of boiling water. The vegetable cooks by contact with the steam produced by the boiling water. You should steam foods until they are crisp-tender; crisp enough to retain good taste and texture and tender enough to sink your teeth into.

Pressure cooking allows you to cook vegetables more quickly than by any other method since it is the only one to allow internal temperatures to reach well above the 212°F mark. One scientific report states that there is no significant advantage to pressure cooking over ordinary steaming. Another report, however, found that pressure cooking is "better than the other methods, because it leads to maximum retention of minerals, ascorbic acid, and riboflavin."[14] Regardless of which report is more accurate, both steaming and pressure cooking are good methods of preparation.

Quick frying, whether by French sautéing or Chinese stir frying, is another excellent way to cook vegetables and preserve maximum nutritional levels. Since no water is used, there is virtually no leaching. And since the process is quick, there is very short exposure to heat, which

Tips on Cooking the Popular Potato

Here are a few words to the nutrition-wise cook in regard to the most popular and widely used of vegetables—the potato. Potatoes, fortunately, are reluctant to give up their vitamin C, as well as other vitamins and minerals. One study showed that whole, unpared Katahdin potatoes, covered and boiled for 40 minutes, retained up to 99.4 percent of their ascorbic acid.[15] Baked potatoes, as well, retain the bulk of their nutrients. Potatoes are susceptible to vitamin and mineral loss by water leaching, however. If they are peeled or cut up in any way, nutrient losses are rapid and severe. A good visual guide is the color of the water after boiling. If it is virtually clear, as it should be when potatoes are boiled whole, then you have lost relatively few vitamins and minerals. But if it is yellowish, as it will be if they are chopped or diced, you will then know that you are pouring vitamins and minerals down the drain.

means less thermal destruction of vitamins and minerals. Nutritionally, quick frying ranks right up there with steaming and pressure cooking.

You can also use a double boiler for nearly waterless cooking. First, put a few inches of water into the bottom pot and bring it to a boil. Then put a few tablespoons of water in the top part, and bring it to a quick boil over another burner. Quickly add the vegetables to the top container, cover, and steam them for just a minute. To finish cooking, place the top container containing the vegetables, still covered, over the bottom half. The steam generated in the bottom container will quickly bring the vegetables to the crisp-tender stage with virtually no loss of nutrients by leaching.

Microwave cooking has been found comparable to the other recommended methods in terms of preserving optimum amounts of vitamins and minerals. Again, however, there are safety questions surrounding microwave ovens.

Cooking techniques aren't the only factors that affect nutrition. Cooking utensils can also have an effect on the nutritional value of foods cooked in them. Unlined copper pots are probably the worst culprits when it comes to affecting foods. Foods that come in direct contact with uncoated copper can have their taste and appearance altered, and it has been reported that their vitamin C is destroyed as well. Also, the acids in fruits and vegetables can combine with the copper to form toxic substances. This doesn't mean that *all* copper pots are unsafe (good news for serious cooks who know that copper gives the best heat distribution). Your best bet is to avoid the use of unlined copper pots and to use only lined cookware. If the lining becomes so worn that the copper is exposed, have the pot relined. In any case, avoid letting your food come in contact with copper.

Over the years, there has been some concern about the safety of using aluminum cookware. It is generally believed by medical researchers that the small amount of aluminum that leaches into food does not represent a health hazard. Some individuals with an extreme sensitivity to aluminum might develop a reaction, but that would be a rare occurrence.

In general, the cooking utensils to use with a clear conscience are made of stainless steel, glass, cast iron, and enamel.

Leftovers, for obvious reasons, should be avoided whenever possible. Cooked foods are even more susceptible to nutrient loss than are raw foods, since their cells have been broken down already during the cooking process. If you store a dish of steamed broccoli in the refrigerator for a few days, do not expect to find much nutritional quality left after you reheat it and serve it the second time. Don't cook more vegetables than will be eaten in a single sitting. If you want to provide a safety margin of food so that nobody leaves the table hungry, be generous in preparing other foods. Treat your cooked vegetables as one-time treasures.

A last word for the kitchen concerns the use of baking soda and salt. A pinch of baking soda added to a pot of cooking beans will help keep the beans bright green and lively looking. It will also double the rate at which the vitamin B complex is lost. Salt added to vegetables, in addition to contributing to already dangerous levels of sodium in the diet, acts to draw moisture more quickly out of vegetable tissue cells. This serves to quicken the loss of all vitamins and minerals during cooking. We all get far more salt than we need from other foods without adding it to our own vegetables which are, in themselves, delicious enough.

Sodium Content of Fresh Vegetables vs. Commercially Processed Vegetables

Vegetable	Sodium (mg per ½ cup)		
	Fresh	Frozen	Canned
Asparagus	1.0	1.0	288
Lima beans	1.0	86.0	292
Snap beans	2.5	0.5	282
Beets	36.5	...	200
Broccoli	8.0	14.0	...
Brussels sprouts	8.0	11.0	...
Carrots	25.5	...	183
Cauliflower	5.5	9.0	...
Collards	18.0	13.5	...
Corn	trace	1.0	248
Kale	23.5	3.5	...
Mustard greens	12.5	7.5	...
Peas	0.5	50.0	115
Spinach	45.0	53.5	274
Winter squash	1.0	1.0	...
Sweet potatoes	13.0	...	61
Tomatoes	5.0	...	156

SOURCES: *Adapted from* Nutritive Value of American Foods in Common Units, *Agriculture Handbook No. 456, by Catherine F. Adams (Agricultural Research Service, U.S. Department of Agriculture, 1975) and "Sodium and Potassium," by George R. Meneely and Harold D. Battarbee,* Nutrition Reviews, *August, 1976.*

CHAPTER 7

Growing for Nutrition

After reading through the first six chapters of this book, you may have decided that amaranth, lentils, and kale are crops you should be growing because of the significant nutrient contributions they can make to your family's diet. But suppose you've never raised any of those particular crops before—how do you know whether your climate is okay, whether the type of soil you've got is suitable, or even whether the season is long enough for the crop to mature? This chapter is meant to answer those types of questions by giving you a rundown of the pertinent cultural characteristics for 76 individual fruits, nuts, and vegetables. You'll find out what each crop needs in the way of growing range, soil requirements, water and nutrient needs, and harvest and storage procedures. You'll also see how long you must wait before you can start harvesting and putting food on the table (weeks in the case of some vegetables, years for some fruits and nuts). A four-star ranking system gives you a handy nutrient profile for each crop so you can compare the relative nutrient strengths and weaknesses of various crops at a glance. (The Key to Nutritional Highlights that follows explains the four-star rankings.)

This chapter isn't intended to be a comprehensive, how-to-grow-it gardening guide. Instead, it is meant to help you make enlightened choices that can significantly raise the nutritional value of your garden. You

137

should refer to this chapter often while you're still in the planning stage.

Once you have some idea of what it takes to grow a particular crop, you'll be better able to match it to your unique set of gardening conditions. The information given here will help you make the final decision of whether or not to include a given crop in the garden. It can also help you figure out the most nutritious succession planting schemes: compare the nutritional highlights, temperature preferences, and days to harvest of various annual vegetables to see how you can keep the garden producing nonstop, from one end of the season to the other. If you're contemplating planting fruit trees and berry bushes, you can quickly compare their relative nutritional merits to see which kinds of fruit match your nutrient criteria and which kinds will thrive in your particular area.

KEY TO NUTRITIONAL HIGHLIGHTS

★★★★ Exceptionally rich source
★★★ Very rich source
★★ Rich source
★ Above-average source

Almonds
Prunus dulcis
Rosaceae

NUTRITIONAL HIGHLIGHTS
Protein★★
Calcium★★
Phosphorus★★★★
Iron★
Riboflavin★★★★
Niacin★★
Modest amounts of potassium and thiamine.

Growing Range: Limited to areas where winters are mild and spring frosts absent. Almost as hardy as the peach but more susceptible to spring frosts because the almond tree blooms earlier than the peach.

Soil Requirements: Provide a sandy and well-drained soil with a neutral or slightly alkaline pH.

Culture: Prepare soil deeply when planting trees. Work compost into soil every autumn, or grow cover crops among trees.

Harvest and Storage: Trees begin to bear in 3 or 4 years and should be in full production in 12 years. Harvest nuts in autumn when those in center of tree are ripe. After harvesting, shell and dry nuts for storage.

Amaranth
Amaranthus
tricolor
Amaranthaceae

NUTRITIONAL HIGHLIGHTS
Protein★
Calcium★★★★
Iron★★★★
Potassium★★★
Vitamin A★★★
Riboflavin★★★
Niacin★★
Vitamin C★★★★
Modest amounts of thiamine.

Growing Range: Suitable for all temperate areas but does best in climates with hot and humid weather.

Temperature Preference: Grows best at 70° to 90°F. Sensitive to frost.

Soil Requirements: Loose, rich, well-drained soil with good supply of nitrogen is best. Not particularly sensitive to pH.

Culture: Sow outdoors when all danger of frost is past, or start plants indoors three weeks before frost-free date. Plant outdoors when danger of frost is past. Thin to 6 inches between plants in beds or rows. No mulching needed between plants because of quick growth.

Harvest and Storage: Ready to harvest in an average of 70 days. Harvest leafy rosettes at top of plant as they appear, when plant is 4 to 6 inches tall. Continue to harvest rosettes as they develop again and again through growing season. Freeze like spinach.
• For a discussion of amaranth's nutritional attributes, see Superior Vegetables and Fruits in chapter 2.

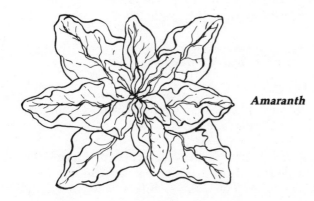

Amaranth

Apples
Malus pumila
Rosaceae

NUTRITIONAL HIGHLIGHTS
Not superior in any element.

Growing Range: There are varieties suited to all temperate zones.

Soil Requirements: Any average garden soil is adequate. Apples prefer pH range of 6.0 to 7.0.

Culture: Many varieties available in dwarf, semidwarf, and standard forms. Trees may be planted in fall or spring (in northernmost regions). Supply ample moisture to roots during first year. Periodic pruning is necessary for best fruit production.

Harvest and Storage: Standard trees start bearing in two to seven years, dwarf trees in two years. Time of harvest is summer to autumn. Harvest when apples are fully ripe for fresh use, before fully ripe for storage. Store in root cellar, basement, or underground pit where temperatures are cool (32° to 40°F) and air is moderately moist. Apples can also be frozen, canned, and dried.
• For a discussion of varieties richest in vitamin C, see box on Superior Apple Varieties in chapter 2.

Apricots
Prunus spp.
Rosaceae

NUTRITIONAL HIGHLIGHTS
Potassium★
Vitamin A★
Modest amounts of protein, riboflavin, niacin, and vitamin C.

Growing Range: Same as for peaches (see entry later in this chapter) except that apricots bloom earlier than peaches and are thus more susceptible to spring frosts. Russian types are hardiest.

Soil Requirements: Average garden soils are suitable. Trees are deep rooted and should not be planted in heavy hardpans.

Culture: Dwarf, semidwarf, and standard forms are available. General culture is same as for peaches except that apricots need far less nitrogen. Excess nitrogen causes immature fruit drop.

Harvest and Storage: Trees start to bear in three years. Time of harvest is summer to autumn. Fully ripe fruit drops from branches. Firm-ripe fruit has changed from green to orange and feels slightly soft when gently squeezed. Apricots to be canned or dried should be allowed to ripen on tree for several days past firm-ripe stage. Fruit can also be frozen.

Asparagus	NUTRITIONAL HIGHLIGHTS
Asparagus *officinalis* Liliaceae	Thiamine★ Riboflavin★ Niacin★ Modest amounts of protein, vitamin A, and vitamin C.

Growing Range: All parts of temperate region are suitable except southernmost areas, where ground does not freeze.

Temperature Preference: Grows best at 60° to 85°F.

Soil Requirements: Any average, well-drained garden soil will do. Good drainage is critical for this perennial crop. Preferred pH is 6.5 to 6.8.

Culture: Dig a trench 18 inches deep and 12 to 15 inches wide, and layer bottom with well-composted manure, leaf mold, peat moss, or combination of these. Plant one-year-old crowns 6 to 10 inches deep several weeks before last spring frost, and gradually fill in trench with topsoil as shoots grow. By midseason, trench should be filled in completely. Keep beds weed free and add thick layer of manure or compost in early autumn to act as mulch and slow-acting fertilizer.

Harvest and Storage: To allow plants time to become established, do not harvest during first two growing seasons. Harvest for two weeks in spring the third season, four weeks the fourth season, and six to eight weeks in subsequent years. Do not cut any season's ferns until following spring. Freezing is best for long-term storage, although spears may also be canned.

Avocados	NUTRITIONAL HIGHLIGHTS
Persea americana Lauraceae	Potassium★★★★ Thiamine★ Riboflavin★★★ Niacin★★★ Modest amounts of protein and vitamin C.

Growing Range: Hardy Mexican-type trees will withstand winter temperatures as low as 18°F without excessive damage. Less hardy Guatemalan types can stand temperatures as low as 24°F. West Indian avocados are the most tender, requiring winter temperatures above 28°F.

Soil Requirements: Good humus content and drainage are key requirements. Not sensitive to pH.

Culture: When ordering trees, be sure variety is suited to area. Plant when all danger of frost has passed. Supply ample moisture all year round, but do not overwater so that puddles form. Excess nitrogen can cause young trees to die back. Little pruning is necessary. Avocados can be grown in greenhouses in containers.

Harvest and Storage: Time of harvest is summer to spring. Determining ripeness is difficult since fruit does not begin to soften until after picked. Fruit that begins to soften five to seven days after harvest was picked at proper time. Some varieties change color to indicate ripeness. Experience and advice of other growers is valuable. Best storage temperature is above 42°F. Avocados can be frozen for long-term storage.

Adzuki Beans
Vigna angularis
Leguminosae

NUTRITIONAL HIGHLIGHTS
Complete nutritional data is not available; adzuki beans are known to be approximately 25 percent protein, ranking with the best of the beans in this category.

Growing Range: Suited to all but very northernmost regions of temperate zone.

Temperature Preference: Tolerate average temperatures from 46° to 82°F. Sensitive to frost.

Soil Requirements: Same as for great northern beans (see entry that follows in this chapter).

Culture: Same as for great northern beans. Do not tolerate waterlogged soil. Adzuki beans are fairly drought resistant.

Harvest and Storage: Harvest while immature for use as snap beans. For dry use, let beans dry on plant. They are ready to harvest in an average of 90 days. Harvest and dry thoroughly indoors before heavy frost. Store in airtight containers in cool, dry place.
• For more information on this crop, see Superior Vegetables and Fruits in chapter 2.

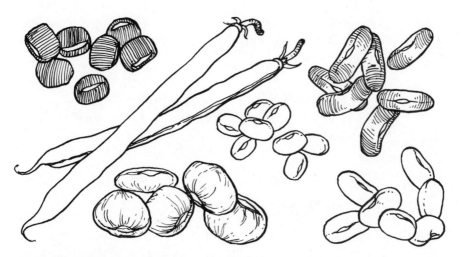

Bean Collection: *Clockwise, from upper left, are adzuki beans, snap beans, navy beans, kidney beans, great northern beans, and lima beans.*

Great Northern Beans	NUTRITIONAL HIGHLIGHTS
Phaseolus vulgaris Leguminosae	Protein★★ Phosphorus★★ Iron★★★ Potassium★★ Thiamine★ Modest amounts of calcium, riboflavin, and niacin.

Growing Range: Suited to all temperate zone areas. Good for short-season areas.

Temperature Preference: Grow best at 60° to 85°F. Sensitive to frost.

Soil Requirements: Need well-drained garden loam, rich in organic matter, phosphorus, and potassium. As legumes, beans fix their own nitrogen on root nodules. The pH range is 6.0 to 7.5.

Culture: Plant seeds into open garden after frost-free date and when soil has warmed to 60° to 65°F. In very short-season areas, start seeds in individual pots three weeks before frost-free date. Use bacterial inoculant powder when planting. Handle roots with care when transplanting, any time danger of frost is past. Feed with potassium in midseason if soil is poor or sandy.

Harvest and Storage: Harvest when seeds have reached full size, for use as green shell beans (around 65 days after sowing). For dry shell beans, wait to harvest until pods are dry and foliage has yellowed, before heavy frost (around 85 days). Dry beans thoroughly indoors and store in airtight containers in cool, dry place.

Green Snap Beans
Phaseolus vulgaris
Leguminosae

NUTRITIONAL HIGHLIGHTS
Modest amounts of protein, thiamine, riboflavin, and niacin.

Growing Range: Suitable for all temperate areas.

Temperature Preference: Grow best at 60° to 70°F. Sensitive to frost.

Soil Requirements: Same as for great northern beans (see preceding entry).

Culture: Same as for great northern beans. Make succession plantings once a week for season-long supply of fresh beans.

Harvest and Storage: Ready to harvest in an average of 48 to 60 days. For use as green snap beans, harvest while pods are young and tender. Can be dried, canned, or frozen.

Kidney Beans
Phaseolus vulgaris
Leguminosae

NUTRITIONAL HIGHLIGHTS
Protein★★★
Phosphorus★★
Iron★★
Potassium★
Thiamine★
Modest amounts of calcium, riboflavin, and niacin.

Growing Range: Same as for great northern beans (see entry earlier in this chapter). Kidney beans need a minimum growing season of 100 days.

Temperature Preference: Grow best at 60° to 70°F. Sensitive to frost.

Soil Requirements: Same as for great northern beans.

Culture: Same as for great northern beans. Kidney beans are easiest of all dry beans to grow.

Harvest and Storage: Same as for great northern beans. Kidney beans require an average of 100 days to reach maturity.

Lima Beans
Phaseolus
lunatus
Leguminosae

NUTRITIONAL HIGHLIGHTS
Protein★★
Calcium★
Phosphorus★
Iron★★
Potassium★
Thiamine★★
Niacin★
Vitamin C★
Modest amounts of riboflavin.

Growing Range: Any region that offers 75 days of warm growing weather will do. Lima beans are very susceptible to even slight chills and may be set back by a cool, rainy period.

Temperature Preference: Grow best at 60° to 70°F. Very sensitive to frost.

Soil Requirements: Same as for great northern beans (see entry earlier in this chapter).

Culture: Same as for great northern beans. Do not plant outdoors until soil temperature has reached a minimum of 65°F.

Harvest and Storage: For green-shell use, harvest when pods are full but before they have begun to yellow (around 65 to 78 days after sowing). For dry storage, see great northern beans. Do not subject to slightest autumn frost.

Navy Beans
Phaseolus
vulgaris
Leguminosae

NUTRITIONAL HIGHLIGHTS
Protein★★★
Phosphorus★★★
Iron★★★★
Potassium★★
Thiamine★★
Modest amounts of calcium, riboflavin, and niacin.

Growing Range: Same as for great northern beans (see entry earlier in this chapter).

Temperature Preference: Same as for great northern beans.

Soil Requirements: Same as for great northern beans.

Culture: Same as for great northern beans.

Harvest and Storage: Same as for great northern beans. Ready to harvest in an average of 85 days.

Yellow Wax Beans
Phaseolus vulgaris
Leguminosae

NUTRITIONAL HIGHLIGHTS
Modest amounts of thiamine and riboflavin.

Growing Range: Do well in all temperate areas.

Temperature Preference: Grow best at 60° to 70°F. Sensitive to frost.

Soil Requirements: Same as for great northern beans (see entry earlier in this chapter).

Culture: Same as for great northern beans. Make succession plantings once a week for season-long supply of fresh beans.

Harvest and Storage: Ready to harvest in an average of 48 to 60 days. For snap use, harvest while pods are young and tender. Can be dried, canned, or frozen.

Beets
Beta vulgaris
Chenopo-
diaceae

NUTRITIONAL HIGHLIGHTS
Greens
Calcium★
Vitamin A★
Thiamine★
Riboflavin★
Modest amounts of protein, iron, potassium, and vitamin C.

Roots
Modest amounts of protein and riboflavin.

Growing Range: Can be grown in all regions but need cool weather as roots reach maturity for best quality.

Temperature Preference: Grow best at 60° to 65°F. Cold tolerant but cannot withstand severe freezing.

Soil Requirements: Suitable for all soils, but beets do best in loose, sandy loam rich in organic matter. Potassium is important for best root development. Nitrogen will spur top growth.

Culture: Sow seeds in open garden two to four weeks before frost-free date. Or start plants indoors four weeks before setting out, which can be done at same time recommended for sowing seeds outdoors. Make succession plantings every two or three weeks. Fall crop may be sown ten weeks before first expected autumn frost. Beets are suitable for wide rows and double rows. Thin plants carefully. Preserve even moisture throughout growing season with thick mulch. Rich soil and good moisture will lead to quick and tender root development. Hot weather causes bolting and woody roots.

Harvest and Storage: Harvest greens anytime they reach usable size. Roots are ready to harvest in an average of 56 to 70 days. Dig roots when they are still small (1½ to 3 inches). Freeze greens for best nutritional retention. Fall-harvested roots can be layered in sand or peat moss and stored at 32° to 40°F under fairly moist conditions. Roots can also be frozen or canned.

Blackberry	NUTRITIONAL HIGHLIGHTS
Rubus spp. Rosaceae	Modest amounts of vitamin C.

Growing Range: At least a dozen different varieties (some variously known as boysenberry, dewberry, loganberry, and youngberry) are suitable for various areas of the temperate zone.

Soil Requirements: All average soils are suitable except very acid soils.

Culture: Propagate from root cuttings. One-year-old cuttings planted 1 to 3 feet apart will fill in a row within two years. Pruning is important for good yields and disease prevention. Mulch will increase yields greatly.

Harvest and Storage: Bushes start bearing when one year old. Harvest berries in summer when fully ripe. This is several days after berries blacken, when they separate easily from the bush. Freezing is best for preserving quality, although berries can also be canned or dried.

Blueberry	NUTRITIONAL HIGHLIGHTS
Vaccinium spp. Ericaceae	Modest amounts of vitamin C.

Growing Range: There are varieties suitable for all parts of temperate zone. Highbush types are suited to areas from Florida to Maine and Michigan. Rabbiteye types are better suited to hot and dry conditions.

Soil Requirements: Any acid soil with good drainage is suitable. Ideal pH is 4.2 to 5.5.

Culture: Plant either rabbiteye or highbush types in spring as two-year-old plants. Work acid materials into soil before planting, and mulch throughout year with acid materials. No other fertilizer is required. Plant highbush plants 6 feet apart, rabbiteye plants 7 to 8 feet apart. Follow regular pruning schedule.

Harvest and Storage: Bushes start bearing when one to two years old. Time of harvest is summer. Berries turn blue when approaching ripeness. For best quality, begin to harvest six days after first berries have turned blue, and continue to harvest regularly thereafter. Freezing best preserves fruit quality. Berries can also be canned or dried.

Broccoli
Brassica oleracea
Botrytis Group
Cruciferae

NUTRITIONAL HIGHLIGHTS
Protein★
Calcium★★★
Phosphorus★
Potassium★
Vitamin A★
Thiamine★
Riboflavin★★★★
Niacin★
Vitamin C★★★★
Modest amounts of iron.

Growing Range: Suitable for all temperate zone areas but does best during cool and moist weather.

Temperature Preference: Grows best at 60° to 65°F. Tolerates light frost.

Soil Requirements: Any average garden loam rich in nitrogen is suitable. Add fresh manure in fall, or well-composted manure in spring. Best pH range is 6.7 to 7.2.

Culture: Sow seeds in open garden four to six weeks before frost-free date. Or start plants indoors eight weeks before frost-free date, and set out seedlings from four weeks before to three weeks after last frost. Two-week succession plantings will produce steady supply of main heads. For rapid growth, mulch heavily and sidedress once or twice during season with compost, manure, or manure tea. Assure good moisture and cool soil temperature during growing season with heavy mulch.

Harvest and Storage: Ready to harvest in an average of 55 to 78 days after transplanting. Cut main head close to base to encourage development of smaller side shoots, which may continue to form up until killing frost. Harvest heads before yellow florets appear. Heads will keep in refrigerator for up to two weeks but with rapid loss of nutrients. Freezing is best for long-term storage, although broccoli can also be canned.

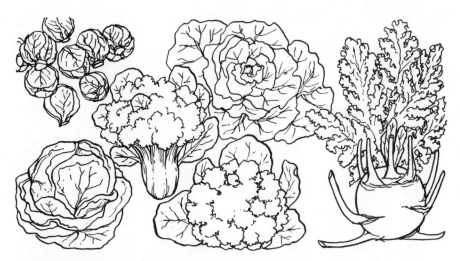

Cabbage Family Portrait: *Clockwise from upper left, these crops include Brussels sprouts, collards, kale, kohlrabi, cauliflower, broccoli, and cabbage.*

Brussels Sprouts *Brassica oleracea* Gemmifera Group Cruciferae	**NUTRITIONAL HIGHLIGHTS** Calcium★ Riboflavin★ Vitamin C★★★ Modest amounts of protein, potassium, thiamine, and niacin.

Growing Range: Require long growing season with cool temperatures, especially as plants mature. In southernmost areas, grow as fall or winter crop.

Temperature Preference: Grow best at 60° to 65°F. Can withstand fairly heavy autumn frosts.

Soil Requirements: Need rich, well-drained soil well supplied with organic matter. Plants do better on heavy soils than on sandy soils and need good supplies of potassium and phosphorus. The pH range is 6.0 to 6.8.

Culture: Sow seeds into open garden 10 to 12 weeks before frost-free date. In very short-season areas start plants indoors 6 weeks before setting out. Transplant at same time as recommended for outdoor seed sowing. Use cutworm collars. Mulch heavily to provide even soil moisture and even soil temperature. Heavy winds may topple plants in late season if staking is not provided. Do not cultivate close to plants.

Harvest and Storage: Ready to harvest in an average of 90 to 100 days after transplanting. Cut sprouts from stalks when they reach good size (1 to 1½ inches). Sprouts mature from bottom of plant upwards. Remove yellowed leaves from stalk to encourage sprout development. Quality of sprouts is improved by first autumn frosts. Store sprouts at 30° to 42°F under moist conditions for up to five weeks. Freeze or can for long-term storage.

Cabbage
Brassica oleracea
Capitata Group
Cruciferae

NUTRITIONAL HIGHLIGHTS
Vitamin C★★

Growing Range: Cool-weather crop suited to all areas of temperate zone. In southernmost regions, grow only as fall or winter crop.

Temperature Preference: Grows best at 60° to 65°F. Can withstand temperatures as low as 20°F.

Soil Requirements: Rich garden loam or muck soils are best. Sandy soils may offer insufficient moisture for this crop's heavy demands. Incorporate copious amounts of well-composted manure 12 inches into soil before planting. Quick and tender growth depends on adequate soil moisture and nutrient supply. Best pH is 6.0 to 6.8; where clubroot is recurring problem, raise pH to 7.2.

Culture: Begin early crop indoors three weeks before last average spring frost and set out plants on frost-free date. Sow seeds of late crop directly into garden rows one month after planting early crop. Sidedress with compost three weeks after setting out, or apply manure tea every three weeks during growing season. Mulch heavily for even soil moisture and to keep down weeds. Supply nitrogen if leaves begin to yellow.

Harvest and Storage: Heads are ready for harvest anytime they are large and solid enough to make effort worthwhile, anywhere from an average of

62 to 120 days after transplanting. Small heads are richer in vitamin C than large ones because of their lower water content. Cut head at base and remove as few outer leaves as possible since outer leaves are richer in vitamin C. Use early crop as harvested. Late crop can be stored for up to six months at 32° to 40°F under moderately moist conditions. For long-term storage, can or freeze.

Carrots	NUTRITIONAL HIGHLIGHTS
Daucus carota var. *sativus* Umbelliferae	Vitamin A★★★★ Modest amounts of potassium, thiamine, riboflavin, and niacin.

Growing Range: Suitable for all temperate zone areas. In north, carrots are grown from early spring through autumn. In southernmost regions, they are commonly grown in fall, winter, and spring.

Temperature Preference: Grow best at 60° to 65°F. Can withstand summer heat as well as light frosts.

Soil Requirements: Light, sandy loam with good drainage is ideal. Best pH range is 6.0 to 6.8. Fine and deep soil preparation is important for best crops, especially when planting long varieties such as Imperator. Add phosphorus and potassium fertilizer but not nitrogen, since excess will cause overly abundant top growth and misshapen roots.

Culture: Sow seeds directly into open garden beginning 4 weeks before frost-free date. Continue with succession plantings every 3 weeks for season-long supply. Or use as succession crop following early cabbage or beans, for example. For winter storage crop, sow seed 12 weeks before first expected autumn frost. Carrots are suitable for wide and double rows. Do not overseed, in order to avoid painstaking thinning later on. Mulch heavily to assure even soil moisture throughout growing season.

Harvest and Storage: Harvest roots whenever large enough to be of use. Midseason harvest of small roots acts as thinning procedure. Vitamin A increases with maturity of roots. For top vitamin A content, wait to harvest until roots are deep orange color, indicating maximum carotene content. In mild-winter areas, leave carrots in ground under heavy mulch and harvest as needed. In colder regions, store fall crop at 32° to 40°F under moist conditions. Freezing and canning are possible although less desirable than fresh storage.

• For a discussion of the nutritionally superior varieties Imperator and Orlando Gold, see Superior Vegetables and Fruits in chapter 2.

Cauliflower
Brassica oleracea
Botrytis Group
Cruciferae

NUTRITIONAL HIGHLIGHTS
Vitamin C★
Modest amounts of protein, thiamine, riboflavin, and niacin.

Growing Range: Suitable for middle areas of temperate zone, liking neither extreme heat nor cold. Plant early crop to mature before midsummer heat, late crop to mature before frost.

Temperature Preference: Grows best at 60° to 65°F. Does not tolerate temperature extremes.

Soil Requirements: Organic-rich, moisture-holding soil is best. Good drainage is important, but crop will grow well in heavy soils. Good supplies of phosphorus and potassium are important for quick growth. The pH range is 6.0 to 6.8.

Culture: Start early crop indoors 6 to 8 weeks before frost-free date. Transplant to open garden 2 to 4 weeks before frost-free date. For fall crop, sow seeds into open garden 12 weeks before first expected autumn frost. Blanch heads only if browning begins to occur. Blanching of heads leads to vitamin C loss. Fall crops should need no blanching at all.

Harvest and Storage: Ready to harvest in an average of 50 to 125 days after transplanting. Harvest when heads are large and still compact. Fuzzy-looking heads are still of good eating quality. With autumn crop intended for storage, cut stem well below head and keep some of the large leaves cradling head. Fall crops can also be pulled up whole, retaining good part of root structure, and hung upside down in root cellar. Fall crops do best when stored at 32°F under moderately moist conditions. When serving, include some of the small leaves with florets, since the leaves are tasty and rich in vitamin C. For long-term storage of early crop, freezing is best.
• For information on the nutritionally superior variety Early Snowball cauliflower, see Superior Vegetables and Fruits in chapter 2.

Celery
Apium graveolens var. *dulce*
Umbelliferae

NUTRITIONAL HIGHLIGHTS
Not superior in any element.

Growing Range: Requires a long growing season free from extremes of heat and cold.

Temperature Preference: Grows best at 60° to 65°F.

Soil Requirements: Needs an organic-rich soil that holds moisture well. Muck soils are ideal. Good supply of potassium is important. The pH range is 5.8 to 6.7. Prepare soil deeply, to 18 inches.

Culture: Start plants indoors eight weeks before transplanting, and transplant to open garden anywhere from three weeks before to four weeks after frost-free date. In mild-winter climates, seeds may be sown in open garden. Sidedress plants with composted manure or manure tea every three weeks during growing season. Mulch heavily to retain soil moisture and keep down weeds. Cultivating around plants may injure shallow roots. Blanching stalks results in loss of already limited vitamin C content. Higher than average vitamin C values for this crop will be found in darker green stalks and in leaves.

Harvest and Storage: Ready to harvest in an average of 90 to 125 days after transplanting. Cut entire plant at base, or harvest outer stalks as needed. Wilting occurs very quickly after harvest because of high water content of stalks; place stalks in refrigerator as soon as possible. (See a description of the chilling-in-the-field process under When the Fruit Leaves the Vine in chapter 6.) For root-cellar storage, pull up entire plant with as much root system as possible and store it in slightly moist sand at 32° to 34°F. Stalks can be frozen or canned and leaves dried to be used later in soups and stews.

Chard
Beta vulgaris
var. *cicla*
Chenopo-
diaceae

NUTRITIONAL HIGHLIGHTS
Calcium★
Iron★
Vitamin A★★
Thiamine★
Riboflavin★
Modest amounts of protein, potassium, niacin, and vitamin C.

Growing Range: Flourishes in all temperate zone areas. Where winters are not severe, chard may overwinter and produce second crop in spring.

Temperature Preference: Grows best at 60° to 65°F. Tolerates both very hot weather and some frost.

Soil Requirements: Any rich soil with adequate drainage is suitable. Additions of balanced compost will spur quick, lush growth. Best pH range is 6.0 to 6.8.

Culture: Sow seeds in open garden two to four weeks before the frost-free date. For earlier crop, start plants indoors four weeks before setting out, and transplant at same time as seeds would be sown outdoors. Bolting is caused by lack of moisture, not by excessive heat. Assure good soil moisture by mulching. In poor soils, apply manure tea several times during growing season.

Harvest and Storage: Ready to harvest in an average of 50 to 60 days. For top vitamin C content, harvest darker green, outer leaves as needed throughout season. When these are removed, next set of leaves will then gain in vitamin C content by exposure to sun. Freeze or can for long-term storage.

<table>
<tr><td>

Sour
Cherries
Prunus cerasus
Rosaceae
</td><td>

NUTRITIONAL HIGHLIGHTS
Modest amounts of vitamin A.
</td></tr>
</table>

Growing Range: Suitable for most temperate zone areas. Sour varieties are generally more hardy than sweet cherry varieties. Bush types are more hardy than standard tree types.

Soil Requirements: Any average garden soil will do. Cherries prefer pH range of 6.0 to 8.0.

Culture: Many varieties available in dwarf, semidwarf, standard, and bush forms. Trees may be planted in fall or (in northernmost regions) spring. Supply ample moisture to roots during first year. Periodic pruning is necessary for best fruit production.

Harvest and Storage: Trees start bearing two to three years after planting. Time of harvest is summer. Pick when fully ripe but before fruit begins to soften. Freeze or can for long-term storage.

<table>
<tr><td>

Sweet
Cherries
Prunus avium
Rosaceae
</td><td>

NUTRITIONAL HIGHLIGHTS
Modest amounts of riboflavin.
</td></tr>
</table>

Growing Range: Same as for peaches (see entry later in this chapter) except that sweet cherries may bloom a few days earlier, thus subjecting blossoms to early spring frosts.

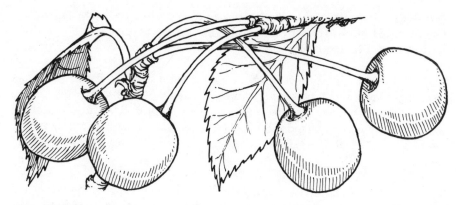

Sour Cherries

Soil Requirements: Same as for sour cherries (see preceding entry).

Culture: Same as for sour cherries.

Harvest and Storage: Same as for sour cherries. Trees start bearing when three to four years old. Time of harvest is summer.

Chinese Cabbage	NUTRITIONAL HIGHLIGHTS
Brassica rapa Pekinensis Group (wong bok) Chinensis Group (bok choy) Cruciferae	Modest amounts of vitamin C.

Growing Range: Cool-season crop, suited to all temperate zone areas. Cool temperatures are especially important as crop comes to maturity. In short-season areas, plant in mid to late summer to harvest as autumn crop; in warm climates, plant as winter or early-spring crop. Suitable for autumn cold-frame growing in north.

Temperature Preference: Grows best at 60° to 65°F. Can withstand temperatures as low as 20°F.

Soil Requirements: Not particular as to soil type, but adequate moisture is essential for quick growth. Good supply of organic matter will result in better crops. The pH range is 6.0 to 6.8.

Culture: For an early spring crop, start plants indoors 8 weeks before frost-free date, and transplant to open garden 4 weeks later. Fall crop is usually more successful since it is less likely to bolt. Sow into garden 12 weeks before first expected fall frost. For even soil moisture, mulch during hot and dry periods. Remove mulch when cool autumn temperatures arrive.

Harvest and Storage: Heading types (Pekinensis Group) can be harvested whenever of usable size; pull up entire plant and retain as many of the outer leaves as possible for maximum vitamin C content. Leaf types (Chinensis Group) can be treated as cut-and-come-again crops; harvest outer leaves as needed. In all varieties, highest vitamin C content is in outer leaves. Heads can be stored for up to four months at 32° to 40°F under moist conditions.

Collards
Brassica oleracea
Acephala
Group
Cruciferae

NUTRITIONAL HIGHLIGHTS
Calcium★★★★
Vitamin A★★★
Thiamine★
Riboflavin★★
Niacin★
Vitamin C★★★
Modest amounts of protein and potassium.

Growing Range: Suitable for all temperate zone areas. Commonly grown in warm climates because they are slow to bolt in heat, but best quality is achieved in cooler climates.

Temperature Preference: Grow best at 60° to 65°F. Can tolerate moderate frost (25°F).

Soil Requirements: Any average, well-drained garden soil is suitable. Incorporate plenty of composted manure before planting, to feed shallow roots. The pH range is 5.5 to 6.8, with an ideal of 6.0.

Culture: Sow seeds directly into open garden 4 weeks before frost-free date or anytime thereafter. For early crop, start plants indoors 4 weeks before setting them out. They can be transplanted anywhere from 4 weeks before to 2 weeks after the frost-free date. For fall crop, seed outdoors 10 to 13 weeks before first expected fall frost. When plants are 6 inches tall, sidedress with manure tea. Repeat applications every 3 weeks for best crop development. If compost is used to sidedress, be careful not to injure shallow roots. Mulch to preserve soil moisture and prolong fall harvest.

Harvest and Storage: Ready to harvest in an average of 70 to 85 days. Inner leaves are more succulent, but darker green outer leaves are richer in vitamin C. Harvest outer leaves before they become tough, or harvest entire plants as needed. Whole plants can be stored for up to three weeks at 32° to 40°F. Freeze or can for long-term storage.

Corn
Zea mays var.
Gramineae

NUTRITIONAL HIGHLIGHTS

Niacin★
Modest amounts of protein, thiamine, and riboflavin.

Growing Range: Grows throughout temperate zone except in northernmost regions that cannot offer the 70- to 100-day growing season required.

Temperature Preference: Grows best at 60° to 75°F. Very sensitive to frost.

Soil Requirements: Any average, well-drained loam will do. Corn requires good nitrogen supplies. Recommended pH is 6.0 to 6.8.

Culture: Sow early varieties directly into open garden around date of last average spring frost. Plant mid- and late-season varieties 10 to 14 days later. Stagger plantings for long-term supply of fresh ears. In northernmost areas, start plants indoors in individual containers two weeks before setting out, which can be done two weeks after frost-free date. Be careful not to disturb roots. Apply mulch when seedlings are 6 to 8 inches tall. Assure adequate soil moisture throughout growing season.

Harvest and Storage: Ready to harvest in an average of 70 to 100 days. Ears are at peak of ripeness when milk spurts out as kernel is pierced with fingernail. Process corn for table use or long-term storage as quickly as possible after harvest. Delay causes quick deterioration of quality as sugars are converted to starches. For long-term storage, freeze, can, or dry. For short-term storage, keep in husks in refrigerator.

Cowpeas (also called blackeye peas) *Vigna unguiculata* Leguminosae	**NUTRITIONAL HIGHLIGHTS** Protein★★ Phosphorus★★ Iron★ Potassium★ Thiamine★★★★ Riboflavin★ Niacin★★ Modest amounts of vitamin C.

Growing Range: Warm-weather crop, suitable for any area that offers long, hot summers.

Temperature Preference: Grow best at 60° to 75°F. Very sensitive to frost.

Soil Requirements: Most soils are suitable, except those that lack good drainage. Supply phosphorus and potassium. Excess nitrogen impedes good seed formation. Best pH range is 6.5 to 7.0.

Culture: Same as for great northern beans (see entry earlier in this chapter). Can withstand drought better than any other bean.

Harvest and Storage: For use as snap beans, harvest pods while they are young and tender. For green-shell use, harvest when pods are full but before they have begun to yellow (around 65 to 85 days). For dry use, treat as described for great northern beans. Green shell beans can be frozen or canned.

Cucumbers *Cucumis sativus* Cucurbitaceae	**NUTRITIONAL HIGHLIGHTS** Not superior in any element.

Growing Range: Do well in all temperate zone areas that are not prone to long spells of cool, damp weather.

Temperature Preference: Grow best at 65° to 75°F. Very sensitive to frost.

Soil Requirements: Any average garden loam with good supply of organic matter is suitable. In sandy soils, assure continuing soil moisture for good fruit development. Add compost to soil before planting.

Culture: Sow seeds directly into ground one or two weeks after frost-free date. In short-season areas, start seeds indoors in individual containers two to three weeks before transplanting, which can be done anytime after last frost date. Handle seedlings gently since their roots are very shallow and easily disturbed. Apply mulch as soon as soil has warmed up. Assure even soil moisture throughout growing season.

Harvest and Storage: Ready to harvest in an average of 48 to 72 days. Harvest pickling types every day to get fruits of good pickling size. Harvest slicing types as needed, but do not allow fruits to mature to yellow stage on vine. Remove all misshapen and overgrown fruit in order to encourage further fruit production. Pickled cucumbers, although a traditional treat, offer little nutritional value and are apt to contain high amounts of sodium. Other than pickling, there is no practical way to store cucumbers for the long term.

Dandelion Greens
Taraxacum officinale
Compositae

NUTRITIONAL HIGHLIGHTS
Calcium★★★★
Iron★
Vitamin A★★★★
Thiamine★
Riboflavin★★
Modest amounts of protein, potassium, and vitamin C.

Growing Range: Thrive in all temperate areas.

Temperature Preference: Grow best at 60° to 65°F.

Soil Requirements: Not particular as to soil type.

Culture: Dandelions, freely growing wild herbs, are seldom cultivated in North America, although they have been grown for centuries in parts of Europe and Asia as medicinal herbs. North American gardeners don't have to make room for them in the garden plot since dandelions can be gathered easily in fields.

Harvest and Storage: Do not gather in public parks or other areas where herbicides may be used for dandelion control. Pick leaves when young and tender, before flowers appear. Cook as a potherb or use raw in salads. Can or freeze for long-term storage.

Eggplants
Solanum melongena
var. *esculentum*
Solanaceae

NUTRITIONAL HIGHLIGHTS
Modest amounts of protein, thiamine, riboflavin, and niacin.

Growing Range: Suited to warmer areas of temperate zone. Early-maturing varieties may be grown in northern regions so long as warm growing weather permits.

Temperature Preference: Grows best at 70° to 85°F. Chill sensitive and susceptible to frost.

Soil Requirements: Any average garden soil that is well drained and well supplied with organic matter is adequate. Prepare soil deeply.

Culture: Start plants indoors eight to ten weeks before transplanting. Set out plants two to three weeks after frost-free date. Mulch as soon as soil has warmed up thoroughly. Sidedress with nitrogen and potassium four weeks after transplanting.

Harvest and Storage: Ready to harvest in an average of 50 to 80 days after transplanting. Pick fruits anytime they are large enough to be of use. Fruits that have lost sheen on their skins or have developed brown seeds inside are past their prime. For short-term storage, keep in warm place in high humidity. Can be canned or frozen but with a loss in quality.

Endive
*Cichorium
endivia*
Compositae

NUTRITIONAL HIGHLIGHTS
Modest amounts of calcium, vitamin A, thiamine, and riboflavin.

Growing Range: Does well throughout temperate zone. Cool-weather crop, best grown in fall, winter, or early spring in southernmost areas.

Temperature Preference: Grows best at 60° to 65°F. Frost tolerant; a few light frosts will improve quality of crop.

Soil Requirements: Any average garden soil with high organic matter and good moisture-holding capacity is adequate. Tolerates very acid soils. The pH range is 5.0 to 6.8.

Culture: Sow seeds into open garden 2 to 4 weeks before frost-free date. For an early start, begin plants indoors 4 weeks before transplanting, which can be done at same time as seeds would be sown outdoors. Succession plantings every 2 or 3 weeks will assure steady supply of leaves throughout spring. Start transplants for fall crop 15 weeks before first expected autumn frost, and set out when 4 weeks old. Hot weather causes bolting and poor leaf quality. Blanch heads when plants are 10 to 12 weeks old to tone down bitter taste of leaves. Blanching usually takes 10 to 14 days and destroys vitamin C in the process. As a trade-off, blanch for a shorter period of time to tame some of the bitterness while losing less vitamin C.

Harvest and Storage: Ready to harvest in an average of 85 to 100 days. Entire plant can be harvested at base, but for best vitamin C content, remove outer leaves as needed for salads.

Garden Cress	NUTRITIONAL HIGHLIGHTS

Garden Cress
Lepidium sativum
Cruciferae

NUTRITIONAL HIGHLIGHTS
Vitamin A★★
Riboflavin★
Modest amounts of protein, potassium, niacin, and vitamin C.

Growing Range: Grows well throughout temperate zone. Cool-weather crop, best planted in fall, winter, or early spring in southernmost areas. Quick-growing fall and early-spring crop for cold frames in northern areas.

Temperature Preference: Grows best at 60° to 65°F. Can withstand some frost.

Soil Requirements: Any average garden soil is adequate. The pH range is 6.0 to 6.8.

Culture: Sow seeds directly into open garden as early as two weeks before frost-free date. Make succession plantings every week or two for continuous supply. Remove any flower heads that might appear. Seeds can also be sprouted indoors for winter greens.

Harvest and Storage: Begin to harvest when plants are ten days old, as needed for fresh greens. Harvesting can continue for up to two months under cool temperatures.

Garden Cress

Globe Artichokes *Cynara scolymus* Compositae	**NUTRITIONAL HIGHLIGHTS** Calcium★ Potassium★ Niacin★ Modest amounts of protein, phosphorus, iron, thiamine, riboflavin, and vitamin C.

Growing Range: Traditionally grown as perennials only in cool coastal areas where ground does not freeze in winter. New French varieties (such as Grande Beurre) may now be grown as annuals in colder climates.

Temperature Preference: Grow best at 60° to 65°F.

Soil Requirements: Light, sandy, well-drained, well-composted soil is ideal. Good drainage is essential. Best pH range is 6.0 to 6.5.

Culture: Plants may be grown from seeds, started indoors six weeks before last average frost, but best results are from suckers taken from established plants. Assure ample moisture and fertilizer during growing season. Water is critical as buds appear. In areas without hard winter freezes, plants may be carried over as perennials and will bear for five or more years before they must be replaced. Perennials should not be allowed to bear buds during first season.

Harvest and Storage: Harvesting of buds from perennial plants begins in second season. Time of harvest is summer. Harvest buds when they are full and before, or just after, the bracts show first signs of opening. Store in cool, moderately moist place. Hearts can be pickled, frozen, or canned but with a significant loss of nutrients.

Gooseberry *Ribes rusticum,* *R. hirtellum,* *R. grossularia,* and other species Saxifragaceae	**NUTRITIONAL HIGHLIGHTS** Vitamin C★

Growing Range: Best suited to northern parts of temperate zone. Be sure that varieties are suited to your growing region.

Soil Requirements: Not particular as to soil type so long as good drainage is offered. The pH range is 6.4 to 7.0.

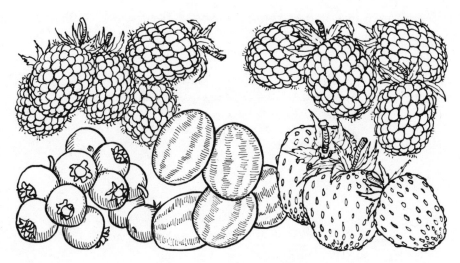

Berry Bunch: *This grouping includes, clockwise from upper left, blackberries, raspberries, strawberries, gooseberries, and blueberries.*

Culture: Start from hardwood cuttings or tip layering in fall or spring (in severe-winter areas). Planting on northern slope will delay spring blooming and perhaps prevent frost damage in southern part of growing range. Follow regular pruning regimen. Keep permanently mulched.

Harvest and Storage: Bushes start bearing when two years old. Time of harvest is summer. Berries are commonly picked while still green and tart, not yet fully mature. Ripe berries are red. Freeze, can, or dry for long-term storage.

Grapefruit
Citrus xparadisi
Rutaceae

NUTRITIONAL HIGHLIGHTS
Vitamin C★★
Modest amounts of thiamine.

Growing Range: Suited to southernmost regions of temperate zone, as well as tropical and semitropical regions. Grows best in hot desert valleys. Withstands moderate frost.

Soil Requirements: Acid soils are best, although the permissible pH range is 5.0 to 7.0. Additions of organic matter will lead to good crops.

Culture: In tropical or semitropical areas, plant young trees anytime. In Florida, planting is done in late winter or early spring; in the Rio Grande Valley of Texas, December and January are favorite planting times. Provide windbreaks in areas with strong or cold winds. Feed annually with organic matter, or grow cover crops in orchard. Most feeder roots are in top 3 feet of soil.

Harvest and Storage: Time of harvest varies according to region and variety. Leave grapefruit on tree until needed. (Fruit must be at least nine to ten months old to be considered mature.) While fruit is awaiting harvest, irrigate trees regularly to retain high juice content of fruit. Both juice and pulp can be frozen or canned.

Concord Grapes *Vitis* spp. Vitaceae	**NUTRITIONAL HIGHLIGHTS** Not superior in any element.

Growing Range: Various varieties of grapes are suited to all parts of temperate zone. Concord grapes are hardy to −15°F. Winter protection needed in northernmost regions.

Soil Requirements: Clay loams, loams, or sandy loams are suitable so long as they offer good drainage and retain warmth. The pH range is 5.5 to 6.7.

Culture: In southern areas, plant dormant vines in fall. Start from one-year-old plants in early spring in northern areas. Choose planting site protected from northwesterly winds and prepare beds the season prior to planting. Mulch for winter protection where needed. Follow careful pruning program for best crops.

Harvest and Storage: Plants start bearing when two years old. Time of harvest is summer. Harvest when fruit is fully ripe, which is when fruit tastes sweet, stems turn brown and shrivel, clusters separate easily from vine, and berry seeds are brown. Remove to cold storage as quickly as possible. Stored in root cellar at 30° to 40°F under moderately moist conditions, fruit will keep up to seven weeks. Juice can be frozen.

Honeydew Melons *Cucumis melo,* Inodorus Group Cucurbitaceae	**NUTRITIONAL HIGHLIGHTS** Potassium★ Niacin★ Vitamin C★ Modest amounts of protein, thiamine, and riboflavin.

Growing Range: Melons do well in any temperate zone area that offers 120 days or more of warm growing weather.

Temperature Preference: Grow best when daytime temperatures average 75°F and nighttime temperatures are a minimum of 55°F. A chill-susceptible crop, but quality of fruit improves as it matures in cool (but not freezing) weather.

Soil Requirements: Light to medium loam, rich in organic matter and capable of holding moisture, is the best. Incorporate copious amounts of well-composted manure before planting. The pH range is 6.0 to 8.0.

Culture: In cooler-climate areas, start seeds indoors in individual containers 10 to 30 days before transplanting. Transplant when soil temperature has reached a minimum of 50°F and daytime temperatures are at a minimum of 80°F. In warmer regions, sow seeds in open garden. Select a sunny spot protected from winds. Apply mulch only when soil has warmed up thoroughly. Assure constant soil moisture. Apply manure tea when fruit sets, and again in two weeks. Potassium, phosphorus, magnesium, and boron are essential to good fruit development. Excess nitrogen can cause soft, misshapen fruit. Keep dry mulch under developing fruit to prevent rotting.

Harvest and Storage: Ready to harvest in an average of 110 days. Fruit is ripe when skin has changed from green to white and has lost its waxy appearance and when blossom end of fruit gives in to thumb pressure. Melons keep from three to four weeks in root cellar at 40° to 50°F, under moist conditions. Mold growth on skin can be inhibited by dipping melon for 30 seconds in water heated to 135°F, then immediately chilling. Peeled melon can also be frozen but with a loss in quality.

Kale
Brassica oleracea
var. *acephala*
Cruciferae

NUTRITIONAL HIGHLIGHTS
Calcium★★
Vitamin A★
Riboflavin★
Niacin★
Vitamin C★★★
Modest amounts of protein and thiamine.

Growing Range: Cool-weather crop suited to northern parts of temperate zone where frosts occur. In southern areas, may be grown as winter crop.

Temperature Preference: Grows best at 60° to 65°F. Languishes in hot weather and tolerates frost very well.

Soil Requirements: Any average garden loam, well drained and well supplied with organic matter, is suitable. Best pH range is 6.5 to 6.8.

Culture: Sow seeds directly into open garden four to six weeks before last average spring frost. Or start plants indoors six to eight weeks before frost-free date, and transplant outdoors anytime from five weeks before to two weeks after frost-free date. When plants are 4 to 5 inches tall, sidedress with manure tea or other nitrogen-rich fertilizer. Keep soil damp but not soggy, and apply mulch when plants are established.

Harvest and Storage: Ready to harvest in an average of 55 days. Use as a cut-and-come-again crop, removing tender young leaves when they are bright green and crisp. Darker green leaves are richest in vitamin C. Use youngest leaves raw in salads; cook older, stronger-tasting leaves as a potherb. In mild-winter areas, mulch crop and harvest as needed throughout winter. Frosts improve quality of leaves. Can also be frozen or canned.
• For a discussion of the nutritionally superior variety Dwarf Scotch kale, see Superior Vegetables and Fruits in chapter 2.

Kohlrabi
Brassica oleracea
Gongylodes
Group
Cruciferae

NUTRITIONAL HIGHLIGHTS
Vitamin C★★
Modest amounts of protein, potassium, and thiamine.

Growing Range: Does well in temperate zone areas that provide at least an 80-day growing season. In northern areas, grow as early-spring and fall crop; in south, grow as fall, winter, or early-spring crop.

Temperature Preference: Grows best at 60° to 65°F. Cool-season crop that tolerates mild frost.

Soil Requirements: Kohlrabi needs sandy loam or loam that is well supplied with organic matter and retains moisture well. Prepare soil finely, to a depth of 8 inches, removing stones and other debris that might impede good root development. Add potassium. Best pH range is 6.0 to 7.0.

Culture: Sow seeds into open garden four to six weeks before frost-free date. In short-season areas, start plants indoors six to eight weeks before transplanting. Transplant anytime from five weeks before to two weeks after frost-free date. Encourage quick and tender growth with good soil moisture and nutrient supply. Do not cultivate close to sensitive roots. Mulch as soon as plants are established.

Harvest and Storage: Ready to harvest in an average of 50 to 60 days. Harvest when bulbs are between 1½ and 2 inches in diameter. Larger bulbs quickly become woody. For short-term storage, keep in refrigerator. In root cellar, maintain 32° to 40°F under moist conditions. Can also be frozen.

Lentils
Lens culinaris
Leguminosae

NUTRITIONAL HIGHLIGHTS
Protein★★★
Phosphorus★★
Iron★★
Modest amounts of potassium, thiamine, riboflavin, and niacin.

Growing Range: Same as for great northern beans (see entry earlier in this chapter). Lentils need longer season than great northern beans.

Temperature Preference: Grow best at 75°F.

Soil Requirements: Suited to sandy, sandy loam, and loam soils. Poorer soils often produce best crops.

Culture: Same as for great northern beans. Not often grown in North America, but culture is not difficult. Lentils do better under drought conditions than in waterlogged soil.

Harvest and Storage: Same as for great northern beans. Ready to harvest in an average of 80 to 130 days.

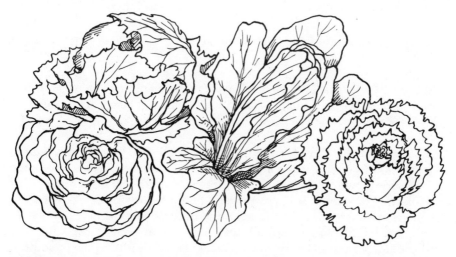

Lettuce Group: *The four main types of lettuce are, clockwise from lower left, butterhead, iceberg, romaine, and leaf.*

Lettuce
Lactuca sativa
Compositae

NUTRITIONAL HIGHLIGHTS

Butterhead
Iron★★★
Potassium★
Modest amounts of protein, calcium, vitamin A, thiamine, riboflavin, and niacin.

Iceberg
Modest amounts of protein, thiamine, riboflavin, and niacin.

Leaf
Calcium★
Iron★
Potassium★
Vitamin A★
Modest amounts of protein, thiamine, riboflavin, niacin, and vitamin C.

Romaine (cos)
Calcium★
Iron★
Potassium★
Vitamin A★
Modest amounts of protein, thiamine, riboflavin, niacin, and vitamin C.

Growing Range: Cool-weather crop best grown in spring and fall in northern areas of temperate zone. Suitable as fall, winter, or early-spring crop in southern areas.

Temperature Preference: Grows best at 60° to 65°F. Can withstand light frost.

Soil Requirements: Lettuce needs well-drained soil, rich in organic material, that is able to hold moisture. Add well-composted manure for best yields. Recommended pH is 6.0 to 6.8.

Culture: Start head types indoors, four to six weeks before transplanting. Transplant to open garden around frost-free date. Sow leaf types directly into garden, two weeks before frost-free date. Make plantings every three weeks for continuous supply. As warm temperatures approach, plant only bolt-resistant varieties, or stop planting until fall approaches. Start sowing fall crop eight weeks before first expected autumn frost, and make succession plantings every week as long as weather permits. In southern areas, make succession plantings in early fall, and continue as long as cool weather permits. Ideal for cold-frame growing in north. (Iceberg, a crisphead type and the least nutritious of lettuces, is best suited to commercial growing.)

Harvest and Storage: Average days to harvest are 50 to 70 for butterhead, 70 to 85 for head, 40 to 50 for leaf, and 70 to 75 for romaine. Harvest crisphead, romaine, and butterhead types by cutting entire head at base. Harvest leaf types by cutting a few outer leaves at a time as needed for salads. Head types can be kept under refrigeration for short periods only.

Mushroom
Agaricus bisporus
(button
mushroom)
Lentinus edodes
(shiitake
mushroom)
Agaricaceae

NUTRITIONAL HIGHLIGHTS
Riboflavin★★★★
Niacin★★★★
Modest amounts of protein, potassium, and thiamine.

Growing Range: Usually grown indoors under temperatures of 55° to 70°F and humidity of 80 to 85 percent. May also be grown outdoors if these conditions are met.

Soil Requirements: Button mushrooms are grown in medium usually consisting of compost, manure, and shredded straw or hay. Another type, the Oriental shiitake, is grown on logs.

Culture: The first-time grower is advised to purchase a preinoculated kit and follow directions carefully. The growing process is an exacting one.

Harvest and Storage: Ready to harvest in an average of 21 to 28 days. As flushes appear, pick heads as soon as they reach usable size. For long-term storage, mushrooms can be frozen, canned, or dried.

Musk-melons
(also called canta-loupes)
Cucumis melo
Reticulatus
Group
Cucurbitaceae

NUTRITIONAL HIGHLIGHTS
Potassium★
Vitamin A★
Niacin★
Vitamin C★★
Modest amounts of protein, thiamine, and riboflavin.

Growing Range: Same as for honeydew melons (see entry earlier in this chapter) except that muskmelons mature somewhat earlier.

Temperature Preference: Grow best at 65° to 75°F. Sensitive to frost.

Soil Requirements: Same as for honeydew melons.

Culture: Same as for honeydew melons.

Harvest and Storage: Ready to harvest in an average of 85 to 95 days. Fruit is ripe when it separates easily from stem with gentle thumb pressure. Fruit is dead ripe when it separates of its own accord. For short-term storage, keep at 45° to 55°F. Not a good keeper, even for short term. Peeled melon can be frozen but with a loss in quality. For longer harvest, plant several varieties that mature at different times.

Mustard Greens
Brassica juncea
Cruciferae

NUTRITIONAL HIGHLIGHTS
Calcium★★
Vitamin A★
Riboflavin★
Vitamin C★
Modest amounts of protein, iron, thiamine, and niacin.

Growing Range: Cool-weather crop, suitable for all but southernmost areas of temperate zone. In north, grow as spring and fall crop; in warm climates, grow as fall, winter, and early-spring crop.

Temperature Preference: Grow best at 60° to 65°F. Tolerate frost well; flavor of leaves is improved by frost.

Soil Requirements: Not particular as to soil type but responds best to moist soil rich in nutrients. The pH range is 5.5 to 6.8.

Culture: Sow seeds directly into open garden two to four weeks before frost-free date. For early crop, start plants indoors four to six weeks before setting out, which can be done at time seeds would be sown outdoors. Because frost improves crop quality, mustard is best grown as fall crop. Sow seeds directly into garden starting eight weeks before first expected autumn frost. In mild-winter areas, make succession sowings all winter long as weather permits. Mulch crop to keep soil cool and prevent bolting during warm spells. Remove flower heads as they appear.

Harvest and Storage: Ready to harvest in an average of 35 to 55 days. Entire plant can be cut at base. For greater vitamin C content, harvest only outer leaves of each plant as needed. Next-to-outer leaves will then build up greater vitamin C content for next picking. Best-quality leaves are 4 to 5 inches long. Use younger leaves in salads, older ones as potherbs. Freeze or can for long-term storage.

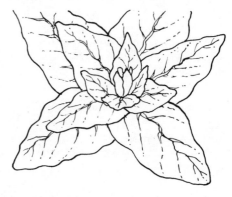

New Zealand Spinach

New
Zealand
Spinach
*Tetragonia
expansa*
Aizoaceae

NUTRITIONAL HIGHLIGHTS
Potassium★★
Vitamin A★
Modest amounts of protein, calcium, iron, riboflavin, niacin, and vitamin C.

Growing Range: Suitable for middle ranges of temperate zone. Requires 90-day-minimum growing season.

Temperature Preference: Grows best at 60° to 75°F. Does not do well in extreme heat; sensitive to frost.

Soil Preparation: Not particular as to soil type, although best crops are grown on moist soil rich in nutrients. The pH range is 6.5 to 7.0. Sensitive to acid soils.

Culture: Sow seeds into open garden one week after frost-free date. Or start plants indoors four to six weeks before transplanting, which can be done two weeks after frost-free date. Pinch growing tips to encourage bushy growth. Keep roots cool and moist with heavy mulch.

Harvest and Storage: Ready to harvest in an average of 70 days. Harvest youngest leaves for best quality. Leaves quickly become too old to be palatable. Use youngest leaves in salads, older ones as potherbs. Freeze for long-term storage.

Okra
Abelmoschus
esculentus
Malvaceae

NUTRITIONAL HIGHLIGHTS
Calcium★★★
Thiamine★★
Riboflavin★★★
Niacin★
Modest amounts of protein, vitamin A, and vitamin C.

Growing Range: Suited to entire temperate zone. Warm-weather crop but will do well in short-season areas that offer two months of warm summer weather.

Temperature Preference: Grows best at 70° to 85°F. Sensitive to frost.

Soil Requirements: Not particular as to soil type. A heavy feeder, it will do best in soil well supplied with nutrients and well drained. Work composted manure 8 inches into soil before planting.

Culture: Sow seeds directly into open garden after frost-free date and once soil temperature has reached a minimum of 60°F. For an early start, begin transplants indoors four weeks before frost-free date and set them out four weeks after frost-free date. For quick growth, sidedress with nitrogen-rich fertilizer every three weeks during growing season. Plants can withstand some drought.

Harvest and Storage: Ready to harvest in an average of 50 to 60 days. Pick pods when only 2 to 3 inches long for best quality. Remove overgrown pods promptly. Use as quickly as possible after harvesting. Freeze or can for long-term storage.

Onions
Allium cepa
Amaryllidaceae

NUTRITIONAL HIGHLIGHTS
Dry
Thiamine★★★

Green
Modest amounts of vitamin A and vitamin C.

Growing Range: All regions of temperate zone are suitable. Daylength determines bulb formation. Be sure to select varieties suited to daylength in your area. Short-day varieties that need 12 hours of light daily are best for southern gardens; long-day varieties that need 13 to 16 hours of light daily are best for northern gardens.

Temperature Preference: Grow best at 55° to 75°F. Tolerate mild frost.

Soil Requirements: Any soil will do except for very heavy clays that will impede bulbs' development. Good drainage is essential. Prepare soil finely and remove stones and other debris. Work in compost, wood ashes, and bone meal. Best pH range, 6.0 to 6.5. Onions are sensitive to overly acid soils.

Culture: Plant sets or seedlings in open garden immediately after frost-free date. In long-season areas, sow seed directly into open garden. In short-season areas, start seedlings indoors four to six weeks before transplanting, which is done immediately after frost-free date. In mild-winter areas, sow seed in fall for scallions in spring. Keep soil well cultivated, weed-free, and moist throughout growing season. Apply mulch at an early stage. Thin as needed throughout season and use thinnings. Pinch off any flower heads.

Harvest and Storage: Harvest and use green onions as needed. For winter storage of dry onions, harvest bulbs after most tops have fallen over and turned brown (around 90 to 150 days after planting). If possible, dry outdoors in sun for three to seven days, then move indoors to warm, dry, shady place to dry for three or four weeks more. Store at 33° to 45°F under dry conditions. Allow for air circulation during storage. Freezing and canning are also possible but less desirable than fresh storage.

Oranges
Citrus sinensis
Rutaceae

NUTRITIONAL HIGHLIGHTS
Calcium★
Thiamine★
Vitamin C★★★
Modest amounts of protein, potassium, riboflavin, and niacin.

Growing Range: Tropical, semitropical, and southernmost parts of temperate zone where ground does not freeze. Can withstand some light frost.

Soil Requirements: Most average garden soils are suitable. Sandy soils must be enriched with organic matter. Good drainage is essential.

Culture: Grow from budded rootstocks. Be sure that variety is suited to your growing area. Dwarf forms are available. Usual planting time is March through May, depending on variety and growing area. Provide windbreaks in areas with strong or cold winds. Feed annually with organic matter, or grow cover crops in orchard.

Harvest and Storage: Color is not always reliable sign of full ripeness. Depend on advice of other growers to determine when fruit has reached maximum juice and sugar content. Valencias in Texas are harvested from

January to May; in California, from March to November; in Arizona, from March to May; in Florida, from March to late June. Florida fruit can be kept eight to ten weeks at 30° to 32°F. California fruit can be kept six to eight weeks at 35° to 37°F. Both juice and pulp can be frozen or canned for long-term storage.

Peaches
Prunus persica
Rosaceae

NUTRITIONAL HIGHLIGHTS
Potassium★
Vitamin A★
Niacin★★
Modest amounts of riboflavin and vitamin C.

Growing Range: Suited to a broad middle range of temperate zone. Where winter temperatures reach as low as −20°F, trees may survive, but fruit will not usually set. Some hardier varieties are now available for northern areas. In southernmost regions, trees might not receive proper length of chilling period (below 45°F for most varieties) necessary to produce blossoms.

Soil Requirements: Any deep, well-drained loam. Excessively sandy soils may not offer sufficient moisture-holding capacity. The pH range is 6.0 to 8.0.

Culture: Be certain that variety is suited to your growing area. Choose sturdy one-year-old stock, 4 to 5 feet tall, with a trunk about ½ inch in diameter. Plant in early spring in northern areas, fall in southern areas. Young trees respond well to nitrogen applications. Thin fruit when it is cherry-size. Water trees during dry spells when fruit is forming. Follow regular pruning schedule.

Harvest and Storage: Trees start bearing when two to three years old. Time of harvest is summer. Highest vitamin content is at full ripeness, when flesh near stem end yields easily to thumb pressure. For long-term storage, freeze, can, or dry.

Peanuts
Arachis hypogaea
Leguminosae

NUTRITIONAL HIGHLIGHTS
Protein★★★★
Phosphorus★★★
Thiamine★
Niacin★★★★
Modest amounts of potassium and riboflavin.

Growing Range: Do well in middle and southern parts of temperate zone with long, warm, and sunny growing seasons.

Temperature Preference: Tolerate average temperatures from 51° to 83°F.

Soil Requirements: Any sandy loam or loam providing good drainage is suitable. Phosphorus and potassium are necessary, but excess nitrogen will lead to poor crop development. Often grown with success in poorer soils. The pH range is 5.0 to 6.0.

Culture: Sow seeds directly into open garden around date of last average spring frost and after soil has reached a minimum of 60°F. Cultivate carefully to avoid root damage. Mulch after runners have buried themselves in soil.

Harvest and Storage: Peanuts are ready when foliage has yellowed, before first autumn frost (around 110 to 120 days after planting). In short-season areas, leave crop in ground until it has matured, after first frosts but before ground freezes. Remove mulch and pull up entire plant to get peanuts adhering to roots, or spade peanuts from ground. Place peanuts on screens or trays and cure them in warm, dry location one month or longer.

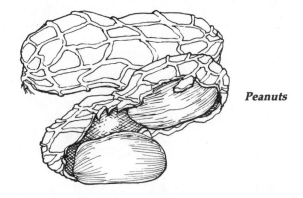

Peanuts

Pears
Pyrus communis
Rosaceae

NUTRITIONAL HIGHLIGHTS
Modest amounts of protein, potassium, and riboflavin.

Growing Range: Middle to upper regions of temperate zone, wherever apples grow. A few varieties are adapted to both warm- and cold-climate areas.

Soil Requirements: Any average, well-drained garden soil is suitable, including heavy loam.

Culture: Many varieties available in dwarf, semidwarf, and standard forms. Trees can be planted in fall or (in northernmost regions) spring.

Supply ample moisture to roots during first year. Periodic but light pruning is recommended for best fruit production.

Harvest and Storage: Standard trees start bearing when three to four years old. Dwarf trees start when two years old. Time of harvest is summer to autumn. Pick fruit two weeks before it is dead ripe and allow it to ripen fully under cool conditions for short-term use. Fruit can be stored for eight weeks or more at 32° to 34°F under moderately moist conditions. Allow stored fruit to ripen fully at room temperatures before using. Pears can also be frozen, canned, or dried.

Peas	NUTRITIONAL HIGHLIGHTS
Pisum sativum	Protein★
Leguminosae	Iron★
	Thiamine★★★★
	Riboflavin★
	Niacin★★★
	Vitamin C★

Growing Range: Cool-weather crop, suited best to northern areas of temperate zone. Peas can also be grown as fall, winter, or early-spring crop in southern regions.

Temperature Preference: Grow best at 60° to 65°F. Excessive heat prevents flower and pod formation. Plants in general tolerate light frost; only blossoms are harmed by low temperatures.

Soil Requirements: Peas grow in any average garden soil except very heavy soil. Soil must be loose, well drained, and well supplied with potassium and phosphorus. The pH range is 6.0 to 7.5.

Culture: Sow seeds directly into open garden 4 to 6 weeks before frost-free date, as soon as ground can be worked. For fall crop, sow seed 12 weeks before first expected autumn frost. Provide supports for climbing varieties. Mulch to keep soil cool and moist.

Harvest and Storage: Ready to harvest in an average of 56 to 75 days. Pick when seeds are fully developed but before pods have begun to deteriorate. Process as quickly as possible after harvesting for best quality. Peas can be frozen, canned, or dried. Peas can also be allowed to dry on vine and treated as described under great northern beans (see entry earlier in this chapter).

Pecans
Carya
illinoinensis
Juglandaceae

NUTRITIONAL HIGHLIGHTS
Thiamine★★★
Modest amounts of protein and riboflavin.

Growing Range: Suited to middle to lower parts of temperate zone. Require hot growing season at least 180 days long.

Soil Requirements: Any garden soil that is deep and well drained is adequate.

Culture: Plant young trees in fall, or start from seed. Be sure that variety is suited to growing area. Be careful not to injure taproot when planting. Fertilize annually with manure, and keep down weeds with mulch.

Harvest and Storage: Trees often begin bearing four to five years after planting. Time of harvest is autumn. In airtight containers, unshelled nuts can be kept at 32° to 38°F for several months. Or, shell and freeze meats.

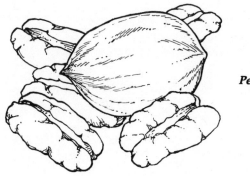

Pecans

Sweet Peppers
Capsicum
annuum
var. *annuum*
Grossum Group
Solanaceae

NUTRITIONAL HIGHLIGHTS
Vitamin C★★★★
Modest amounts of thiamine, riboflavin, and niacin.

Growing Range: Warm-weather crop that grows in temperate areas with 80 days or more of favorable temperatures. Grow as summer crop in northern areas; grow as fall and winter crop only in southernmost areas.

Temperature Preference: Grow best at 70° to 75°F. Very sensitive to chilly weather; plants are stunted and blossoms drop at temperatures below 55°F.

Soil Requirements: Peppers thrive in sandy to average loams, well drained and well supplied with nutrients, including magnesium. The pH range is 6.0 to 7.0.

Culture: Start plants indoors three to five weeks before frost-free date, and transplant to open garden three weeks after frost-free date and when average night temperatures are above 55°F and soil has warmed to a minimum of 60°F. Sow seeds in open garden only in southernmost areas. Keep soil evenly moist throughout growing season. Apply mulch only when soil has warmed up thoroughly.

Harvest and Storage: Ready to harvest in an average of 65 to 80 days after transplanting. Harvest whenever large enough to be of use. Vitamin C content increases with maturity, through red stage. Freeze without blanching for best retention of vitamin C. Peppers can also be canned or dried.

Plums *Prunus* spp. Rosaceae	**NUTRITIONAL HIGHLIGHTS** Modest amounts of thiamine.

Growing Range: Suited to broad middle range of temperate zone, depending on specific variety.

Soil Requirements: Any average garden soil is adequate, including heavier soils as long as they are well drained.

Culture: Plant budded rootstock. Be certain that variety is suited to your growing area. Treat the same as peaches (see entry earlier in this chapter).

Harvest and Storage: Trees start bearing when two to three years old. Time of harvest is summer. Pick when firm-ripe, when fruit has changed color and flesh begins to soften slightly. For short-term storage, keep at 35°F under moderately moist conditions. Plums can be frozen, canned, or dried.

Popcorn *Zea mays* var. *praecox* Gramineae	**NUTRITIONAL HIGHLIGHTS** Modest amounts of protein.

Growing Range: Same as for corn (see entry earlier in this chapter). Requires slightly longer growing season.

Temperature Preference: Same as for corn.

Soil Requirements: Same as for corn.

Culture: Same as for corn.

Harvest and Storage: Ready to harvest in an average of 90 to 120 days. When warm and dry weather permits, allow ears to dry on stalks. If cool and rainy, cut stalks and stack them in sheltered, airy location for a week. Then pick ears, shuck them, and store them in dry location with good air circulation. After a month, test-pop some kernels. If results are unsatisfactory, wait a week or two and try again. When kernels pop well, shell all ears and store kernels in airtight containers placed in cool, dark location.

Potatoes	NUTRITIONAL HIGHLIGHTS
Solanum	Protein★
tuberosum	Phosphorus★
Solanaceae	Potassium★★★★
	Thiamine★★
	Niacin★★★★
	Vitamin C★
	Modest amounts of iron and riboflavin.

Growing Range: Potatoes can be grown in all areas of temperate zone, depending on specific variety.

Temperature Preference: Grow best at 60° to 65°F.

Soil Requirements: Any average garden soil that is loose, well drained, and well supplied with organic matter is suitable. Satisfactory crops are often grown on poorer soils, but plants will respond to phosphorus and potassium applications. Recommended pH range is 5.2 to 5.7. Higher pH encourages scab.

Culture: Plant certified seed potatoes, cutting potatoes so that each piece contains one or two eyes. Plant two to four weeks before frost-free date in well-prepared soil. Keep soil moist but not soggy throughout growing season. Hill up any potatoes that poke through soil surface. Potatoes can also be planted on top of soil under thick layer of mulch.

Harvesting and Storage: For fresh use, harvest tubers as needed, whenever they reach usable size. For winter storage, harvest late varieties as first autumn frosts arrive and as foliage dies down. Potatoes can be left in ground to mature so long as ground does not freeze. Take potatoes indoors to dry for a few hours, then gently brush excess soil away, and store them for one to two weeks in dark, cool, and dry location. Then move to cold location (32° to 40°F) under conditions of high humidity and good ventilation. To increase vitamin C content of stored potatoes, bring into warmer temperatures several weeks before using. (For more details on potato storage, see Vitamins Underground in chapter 6.) Freezing and canning are possible although less desirable than fresh storage.

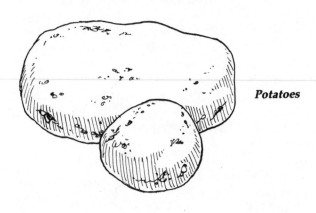

Potatoes

Radishes
Raphanus sativus
Cruciferae

NUTRITIONAL HIGHLIGHTS
Not superior in any element.

Growing Range: Radishes thrive in all ranges of temperate zone. Most varieties require cool temperatures for best development. Grow as an early spring or fall crop in northern areas; grow in fall, winter, or early spring in southern regions. Excessive heat and long daylength cause bolting. There are different varieties for early-, mid-, and late-season plantings.

Temperature Preference: Grow best at 60° to 65°F. Can withstand light frost.

Soil Requirements: Average garden soils that are loose, well drained, and capable of holding moisture are best. Constant moisture supply is essential for quick and tender root development.

Culture: Sow seeds directly into garden in early spring as soon as soil can be worked. Seeds will germinate in soil temperatures above 40°F. Stagger plantings every seven to ten days as long as cool weather permits. In north, sow late varieties ten weeks before first expected autumn frost. In southern areas, sow seeds two months before last expected spring frost, or in fall for winter crop.

Harvest and Storage: Pull up spring crop when roots are young and tender, under 1 inch in diameter (anywhere from an average of 22 to 30 days after planting). Harvest midseason varieties when they are large enough to be of use and late varieties as they mature. These roots are generally ready in around 55 to 60 days. Fall and winter crops may be improved by a few light frosts. Late varieties can be stored at 32° to 40°F under moist conditions.

Raspberries
Rubus spp.
Rosaceae

NUTRITIONAL HIGHLIGHTS

Black
Modest amounts of protein, riboflavin, niacin, and vitamin C.

Red
Modest amounts of riboflavin, niacin, and vitamin C.

Growing Range: Suited to broad middle range of temperate zone, depending on type and variety. Red varieties can withstand more cold, black varieties more heat.

Soil Requirements: Plants do well in any average garden soil that is well drained. Recommended pH is 5.5 to 7.0, with 6.0 ideal.

Culture: Plant virus-free nursery stock in spring, in rows or clumps. Provide supports if recommended for variety. Mulch in spring to conserve soil moisture. Irrigate if necessary during dry periods, especially as fruit forms. Follow recommended pruning schedule. Each cane bears during second year, then dies. Remove dead canes.

Harvest and Storage: Bushes start bearing when one to two years old. Time of harvest is summer and/or fall, depending on variety. Summer varieties are harvested once, while everbearing varieties are harvested twice a season. Harvest every other day during ripening season. Pick berries just before they are dead ripe. Fully ripe berries are very soft and crush and bruise easily. For long-term storage, freezing preserves best taste and quality, although berries can also be canned or dried.

Rhubarb
Rheum
rhaponticum
Polygonaceae

NUTRITIONAL HIGHLIGHTS
Calcium★
Modest amounts of riboflavin.

Growing Range: Grows well in upper regions of temperate zone. Plant must undergo winter dormancy brought on by freezing of crown.

Soil Requirements: Will do well in any average garden soil, although a well-drained sandy loam is best. The pH range is 5.0 to 6.8.

Culture: Plant dormant crowns in fall or early spring. Mulch to conserve soil moisture throughout growing season. Fertilize with well-rotted manure or compost every autumn.

Harvest and Storage: Do not harvest any stalks during first season. Harvest lightly in spring the second year, and make full harvests thereafter. Never harvest more than half the plant in any one season. Pick stalks when they are 12 to 24 inches long. For short-term storage, keep in refrigerator. For long-term storage, freeze or can.

Rutabagas
Brassica napus
Napobrassica
Group
Cruciferae

NUTRITIONAL HIGHLIGHTS
Calcium★
Niacin★
Vitamin C★
Modest amounts of protein, vitamin A, thiamine, and riboflavin.

Growing Range: Suited to all regions of temperate zone that can offer 35 to 50 days of cool growing weather. A single midseason planting is generally made to allow roots to mature in cool fall weather.

Temperature Preference: Grow best at 60° to 65°F. Warm temperatures result in inferior roots. Crop is frost tolerant.

Soil Requirements: Rutabagas thrive in sandy loam or loam that is loose and light to allow for quick root development, able to hold moisture, and rich in nutrients. Incorporate copious amounts of compost for best crops. The pH range is 6.5 to 7.0.

Culture: Plant in midsummer for fall crop, 15 weeks before first expected frost. When thinning plants, use greens in salads.

Harvest and Storage: Harvest any time roots are large enough to be of use (usually ready to harvest in 90 days). Best taste and texture result when plants are subjected to several sharp autumn frosts. Roots will keep up to six months at 32° to 40°F under moist conditions. In mild-winter areas, roots can be kept in garden under heavy mulch, to be harvested as needed. Rutabagas can also be frozen.

Salsify	NUTRITIONAL HIGHLIGHTS
Tragopogon porrifolius Compositae	Modest amounts of protein.

Growing Range: Grows well in middle to upper ranges of temperate zone. Requires 100 or more days to grow to maturity, although roots may be harvested while immature in short-season areas.

Temperature Preference: Grows best at 55° to 75°F. Crop is frost tolerant, and flavor is greatly enhanced by autumn frosts.

Soil Requirements: Needs a loose, well-drained soil able to hold moisture and rich in nutrients. Prepare soil finely to depth of 10 inches. Best pH is 7.0. Lime soil if acid.

Culture: Sow seeds directly into open garden two to four weeks before frost-free date and after soil has warmed to a minimum of 40°F. Mulch to conserve soil moisture. Sidedress monthly with potassium-rich material.

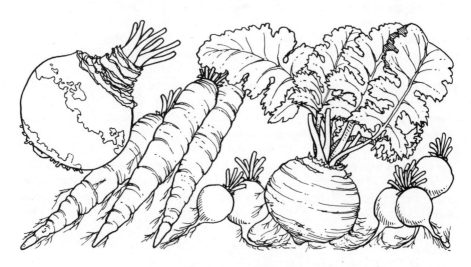

Root Crop Assortment: *From left to right, the crops shown here include rutabaga, salsify, radishes, turnip (with nutrient-rich greens), and more radishes.*

Harvest and Storage: Dig roots anytime they are of usable size (usually ready to harvest in 150 days). Those touched by heavy frost will have best taste and texture. Salsify can be stored in root cellar for up to six months at 32° to 40°F under moist conditions. Roots can be stored in garden under heavy mulch, to be dug as needed. Cut back tops before adding mulch. In northernmost regions where ground freezes deeply, roots can also be stored underground in boxes. Freezing and canning are also possible although less desirable than fresh storage.

Soybeans	NUTRITIONAL HIGHLIGHTS
Glycine max Leguminosae	Protein★★★★ Calcium★ Phosphorus★★★ Iron★★★ Potassium★★★ Thiamine★★★

Modest amounts of riboflavin and niacin.

Growing Range: All but very northernmost regions of temperate zone. Most varieties require 100 or more days of warm growing weather, although there are a few short-season varieties.

Temperature Preference: Tolerate average temperatures from 43° to 82°F.

Soil Requirements: Any average, well-drained garden soil will do. Excess nutrients, especially nitrogen, will result in poor yields. Can be grown successfully on poorer soils; soybeans tolerate soils with low fertility and poor drainage better than most crops. Recommended pH is 6.5 to 7.0.

Culture: Sow seeds directly into open garden after danger of frost is past and when soil has warmed to a minimum of 65°F. Mulch after soil has warmed up thoroughly. Supply water after blossoms have opened if soil is very dry.

Harvest and Storage: For use as green shell beans, harvest when beans are fully developed but before pods have begun to deteriorate (around 85 days after planting). Shell beans can be frozen or canned. For dry storage, harvest when pods are dry but stems are still green. Dry beans thoroughly indoors and store in airtight containers in cool, dry place.

• For a discussion of soybeans' nutritional attributes, see Superior Vegetables and Fruits in chapter 2.

Spinach
Spinacia oleracea
Chenopo-
diaceae

NUTRITIONAL HIGHLIGHTS

Calcium★★
Iron★
Vitamin A★★★
Riboflavin★
Vitamin C★
Modest amounts of protein, potassium, thiamine, and niacin.

Growing Range: Can be successfully grown in any area that offers 50 days of cool temperatures and short daylength. In northern areas, grow as an early spring or fall crop; in southernmost areas, grow as winter crop.

Temperature Preference: Grows best at 60° to 65°F. Can withstand light frost.

Soil Requirements: Any average garden soil is suitable, although spinach does best on sandy loam that is well drained and fairly rich in nutrients. Incorporate well-composted manure into soil for best yields.

Culture: Sow seeds directly into open garden four to six weeks before frost-free date, as soon as soil can be worked. Sow fall crop nine weeks before first expected autumn frost. Stagger plantings a week apart for continuous fresh supply of leaves. Mulch between rows to keep even level of soil moisture. Keep rows free from weeds.

Harvest and Storage: Ready to harvest in an average of 42 to 50 days. Harvest outer leaves only for highest vitamin C content. Next-to-outer leaves will then develop more vitamin C. Spinach can withstand a good amount of fall frost. When killing frost threatens, cut off entire plant at base and freeze for best nutrient retention. If spring crop starts to bolt, harvest and freeze all leaves. Spinach can also be canned.

Squash
*Cucurbita
maxima,
C. mixta,
C. moschata,
C. pepo
var. melopepo,
C. pepo
var. pepo*
Cucurbitaceae

NUTRITIONAL HIGHLIGHTS

Acorn
Potassium★★★
Riboflavin★★
Modest amounts of protein, calcium, iron, vitamin A, thiamine, and vitamin C.

Butternut
Potassium★★★★
Vitamin A★★
Riboflavin★★

Squash— continued	Butternut—continued Modest amounts of protein, calcium, iron, and thiamine.
	Crookneck Riboflavin★ Niacin★ Modest amounts of protein, vitamin A, thiamine, and vitamin C.
	Hubbard Vitamin A★★ Riboflavin★★ Modest amounts of protein, potassium, thiamine, and vitamin C.
	Scallop Riboflavin★ Niacin★ Modest amounts of thiamine and vitamin C.

Growing Range: All squash can be raised in all areas of temperate zone given warm, sunny growing conditions.

Temperature Preference: Grows best at 65° to 75°F. Summer squash is susceptible to frost; winter types can tolerate a few light frosts.

Soil Requirements: Any average garden soil that is well drained, fairly rich in nutrients, and able to hold moisture will support squash. For largest crops, add copious amounts of compost to plot and till to a depth of 12 inches. The pH range is 6.0 to 7.0.

Culture: Sow seeds of both summer and winter types directly into garden when all danger of frost is past and soil temperature has warmed to a minimum of 60°F. In short-season areas, start seeds indoors in individual containers four weeks before setting out, which can be done four weeks after frost-free date. Remove all weeds until soil has warmed up thoroughly, then apply heavy mulch.

Harvest and Storage: Harvest summer types while they are immature and tender, around 40 to 50 days after sowing. Pick regularly for top production and remove overgrown fruits promptly. Summer squash can be frozen or canned. Harvest winter types just before first hard autumn frost, from 85 to 110 days after sowing. A few light frosts will improve taste and texture. Keep all winter squash except acorn type in warm (75° to 85°), moderately dry place for one to two weeks to cure rinds. Then remove to dry location at 50° to 60°F for winter storage. Acorn types should be stored immediately at 32° to 40°F in moist location.

• For profiles of the nutritionally outstanding squash varieties Eat-All, Kuta, and Jersey Golden Acorn, see Superior Vegetables and Fruits in chapter 2.

Strawberries
Fragaria spp.
Rosaceae

NUTRITIONAL HIGHLIGHTS
Vitamin C★★
Modest amounts of calcium, riboflavin, and niacin.

Growing Range: Different varieties are suited for all areas of temperate zone. Be certain that variety you select is suited to your growing area.

Soil Requirements: Average sandy loam or loam, well drained and able to hold moisture, is adequate. Heavy nutrient supply is not necessary. Excess nitrogen will reduce yields. The pH range is 6.5 to 7.2, sometimes depending on specific variety.

Culture: In northern areas, set out young plants in spring. In southern areas, plant in fall. Mother plants bear well for one to two years, but runners produce new plants to take their places. Mulch year-round. Remove old plants and excess runner plants annually.

Harvest and Storage: No harvest is usually taken from new plants during first year, to help them become established. Time of harvest is spring except for everbearing types, which bear in spring and autumn. Harvest every other day when fruit is ripening, picking only ripest berries. Use or process as soon as possible after picking. Freeze for long-term storage.

Sunflower Seeds
Helianthus annuus
Compositae

NUTRITIONAL HIGHLIGHTS
Protein★★★★
Phosphorus★★★★
Iron★★★★
Potassium★
Thiamine★★★★
Niacin★★★
Modest amounts of calcium and riboflavin.

Growing Range: Sunflowers can be grown in any region of temperate zone that offers 80 to 120 days of warm and sunny weather.

Soil Requirements: Any average garden soil that is well drained and fairly well supplied with nutrients will do. Best crops are grown in somewhat sandy soils, well supplied with nutrients and water. The pH range is 6.0 to 8.0.

Culture: Plant seeds directly into open garden around frost-free date. Keep area weed-free until plants are established, and apply mulch when ground has warmed up thoroughly.

Harvest and Storage: When birds begin to eat seeds, they are ripe for harvest, generally 80 to 120 days after sowing. Cut off heads with 1 foot of stem attached, tie into bunches by stems, and hang in warm, airy place to dry. After a month, seeds should come loose quite easily and can be stored in airtight containers.
• For information on the nutritionally superior variety Mammoth Russian sunflower, see Superior Vegetables and Fruits in chapter 2.

Sweet Potatoes
Ipomoea batatas
Convolvulaceae

NUTRITIONAL HIGHLIGHTS
Potassium★
Vitamin A★★★★
Thiamine★
Niacin★
Vitamin C★
Modest amounts of protein, calcium, iron, and riboflavin.

Growing Range: Best crops are grown in regions with long, warm, and sunny summers. Good crops can also be grown in northern areas where summers are shorter but days are longer. Not suitable for northernmost or very cloudy regions.

Temperature Preference: Grow best at 70° to 85°F. Very susceptible to frost damage.

Soil Requirements: Sweet potatoes need sandy loam or loam, light and loose for easy root development. Hardpan soil will lead to poor crops. Rich nutrient supply is not necessary to good crops, although addition of some compost will improve yields. The pH range is 5.5 to 6.5.

Culture: Set out young plants when all danger of frost is past and when soil temperature has reached a minimum of 65°F. Keep after weeds as plants become established. Vigorous vines may make mulching unnecessary. Crop can withstand quite severe drought conditions.

Harvest and Storage: Tubers make major growth spurt during last month of growing season. Harvest immature tubers anytime they are large enough to be of use, but harvest main crop as autumn frosts arrive (around 120 to 150 days after planting). Tubers quickly rot in ground after frosts. After digging, let tubers dry in airy place for an afternoon, then remove to warm and humid place for 10 to 14 days to cure skins. For winter storage, keep at 55° to 60°F under moderately dry conditions. Tubers can also be frozen or canned.
• See the box on Superior Sweet Potato Varieties in chapter 2 for a discussion of vitamin A-rich sweet potatoes.

Tomatoes	NUTRITIONAL HIGHLIGHTS

Tomatoes
Lycopersicon
lycopersicum
Solanaceae

NUTRITIONAL HIGHLIGHTS
Potassium★
Niacin★
Vitamin C★
Modest amounts of protein, vitamin A, thiamine, and riboflavin.

Growing Range: Various varieties are suited to all parts of temperate zone. In extreme north and south regions, be sure that variety is suited to growing area.

Temperature Preference: Grow best at 70° to 75°F. Cannot withstand even light frost.

Soil Requirements: Tomatoes need sandy loam or loam, well drained and well supplied with organic matter. Recommended pH range is 6.0 to 7.0.

Culture: For earliest crops, start plants indoors six to eight weeks before frost-free date, and transplant to open garden about four weeks after that date, when minimum temperature is 55°F. In regions with sufficiently long growing season, sow seed directly into open garden anytime after frost-free date. Mulch when ground has warmed up thoroughly. Stake or cage indeterminate varieties if desired. Sidedress with fish-emulsion solution or weak manure tea only after plants have set fruit.

Harvest and Storage: Ready to harvest in an average of 60 to 90 days after transplanting. Harvest when fruit is a uniform color, before it becomes soft. (With red varieties, red skin color will not develop in temperatures above 86°F, so in southernmost areas, pick when pink.) Use fresh fruit immediately. When heavy frost threatens, harvest all fruit, red and green. Ripen green fruit on sunny windowsill, unwrapped, for best vitamin C content. (For a detailed discussion on how to treat green tomatoes, see

Storing Foods for Quality in chapter 6.) To prevent overripening of already ripe fruit, store at 55° to 60°F. For long-term storage, canning is preferred method although freezing is also suitable.

• For information on the nutritionally superior varieties Caro-Red, Caro-Rich, and Doublerich, see Superior Vegetables and Fruits in chapter 2.

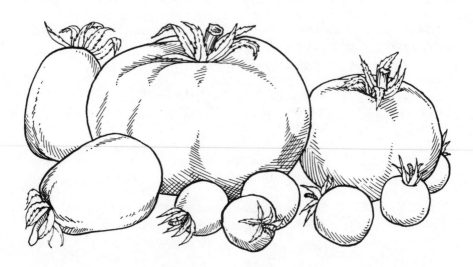

Tomato Medley: *This vegetable comes in several shapes and sizes, as shown from left to right: plum, beefsteak, cherry, and a medium-sized, globe-shaped type.*

Turnips
Brassica rapa
Rapifera Group
Cruciferae

NUTRITIONAL HIGHLIGHTS

Greens
Calcium★★★
Vitamin A★
Thiamine★
Riboflavin★★
Vitamin C★
Modest amounts of protein and niacin.

Roots
Vitamin C★
Modest amounts of calcium, potassium, thiamine, riboflavin, and niacin.

Growing Range: All regions of temperate zone that can offer 35 to 50 days of cool growing weather are suitable. In northern areas, plant in early spring; in southern areas, plant in fall to be harvested in early spring.

Temperature Preference: Grow best at 60° to 65°F. Do not withstand heavy frost well.

Soil Requirements: Turnips thrive in sandy loam or loam that is loose and light to allow for quick root development, able to hold moisture, and rich in nutrients. Incorporate copious amounts of compost for best crops. The pH range is 6.5 to 7.0.

Culture: Sow seeds into open garden in early spring as soon as soil can be worked. Make succession plantings every two or three weeks until hot weather approaches. When thinning plants, use greens in salads. Mulch to keep soil cool and prevent bolting.

Harvest and Storage: Ready to harvest in an average of 40 to 75 days. Dig roots when they are young and tender, 2 to 3 inches in diameter. Pick several leaves from each plant as needed for fresh use in salads. If hot weather causes slightest deterioration of root quality, harvest and preserve entire crop. Both tops and roots can be frozen or canned.

Walnuts
Juglans spp.
Juglandaceae

NUTRITIONAL HIGHLIGHTS

Black
Protein★
Phosphorus★★★★
Iron★
Modest amounts of thiamine.

English
Protein★
Phosphorus★
Modest amounts of thiamine and riboflavin.

Growing Range: Walnuts are suited to most regions of the temperate zone, depending on variety. English walnuts are very demanding as to both soil and climate. Black walnuts are more tolerant and will succeed in northern areas where winter temperatures do not go much below −20°F. When ordering trees, be sure variety is suited to your growing area.

Soil Requirements: Walnuts prefer nutrient-rich loams that are deep, unencumbered by hardpan, and well drained. Black walnuts require 5 feet of unencroached growing area, English walnuts 10 to 12 feet. Recommended pH range is neutral to slightly acid.

Culture: Plant one-year-old grafted rootstock in sunny, protected location. Lawn areas are suitable, since grass will grow under trees, but do not plant black walnut trees near vegetable garden, since a substance in the roots is harmful to tomatoes and other solanaceous crops. Provide adequate soil moisture, especially during and after flowering.

Harvest and Storage: Trees start to bear anywhere from six to ten years after planting. Time of harvest is fall. Shake limbs during ripening period to bring down nuts. Remove husks, wash nuts, dry thoroughly, and store in cool, dry place.

Watercress	NUTRITIONAL HIGHLIGHTS
Nasturtium officinale Cruciferae	Calcium★ Vitamin C★ Modest amounts of vitamin A and riboflavin.

Growing Range: Grows in all regions of temperate zone. Prefers cool weather for best-quality development.

Soil Requirements: Generally grown along banks of cool-water streams. Watercress can also be grown in any soil that is very well supplied with water or in containers supplied with running water.

Culture: Sow seeds along stream bank 6 inches above water level, where soil is constantly moist. Or root supermarket bunches in water and transplant to stream bank. Watercress can also be grown in garden, preferably in container that is frequently flooded with water. Partially shaded area is best, perhaps under large tree.

Harvest and Storage: Ready to harvest in an average of 180 days. Cut tender growing tips as needed for salads or garnish. Remove flower heads as they appear.

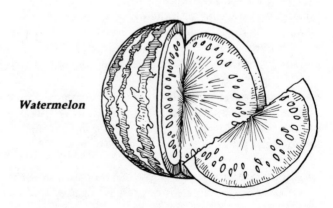

Watermelon

Watermelon
Citrullus lanatus
Cucurbitaceae

NUTRITIONAL HIGHLIGHTS
Iron★★
Potassium★★
Vitamin A★
Thiamine★
Riboflavin★
Niacin★
Vitamin C★
Modest amounts of protein.

Growing Range: Most varieties require long, hot, sunny growing season. Short-season varieties are also available for northern areas. Be certain that variety is suited to your growing region.

Temperature Preference: Grows best at 70° to 85°F. Extremely sensitive to frost.

Soil Requirements: These melons grow in sandy, sandy loam, or light loam soil as long as it is well drained and well supplied with nutrients. Incorporate well-rotted manure or compost into soil to depth of 6 inches, preferably the autumn before planting. For best crops add phosphorus and potassium materials which include wide variety of trace minerals, but do not supply extra nitrogen. The pH range is 6.0 to 7.0.

Culture: Same as for honeydew melons (see entry earlier in this chapter).

Harvest and Storage: Ready to harvest in an average of 75 to 95 days. Harvest when fruit is dead ripe, when a dull "thunk" is recorded upon striking melon with knuckles or when tendril nearest stem has turned brown and dry and stem has become brittle. Experience is the best teacher. (If you take a plug to test for ripeness and melon is not ripe, replace plug and tape up to prevent rot from entering melon.) Peeled melon can be frozen for long-term storage, although at considerable loss in quality.
• For an idea on which varieties contain the most vitamin A, see the box on Superior Watermelon Varieties in chapter 2.

Witloof Chicory
Cichorium intybus
Compositae

NUTRITIONAL HIGHLIGHTS
Not superior in any element when blanched; when not blanched, a good source of vitamin A, vitamin B complex, vitamin C, and several minerals.

Growing Range: Cool-weather crop suitable for all temperate zone areas except southernmost.

Temperature Preference: Grows best at 55° to 75°F. Tolerates light frost.

Soil Requirements: Not particular as to soil type, although roots must be kept moist throughout season. Prepare soil finely to depth of 24 inches and remove all stones and other debris that might interfere with root development. Incorporate compost throughout growing depth. The pH range is 5.0 to 6.8.

Culture: Witloof, unlike other types of chicory, is grown for its roots, which are later forced indoors to provide blanched Belgian or French endive. If not blanched, endive leaves are bitter and virtually unpalatable. If blanched, they surrender their nutritional elements. Sow seeds into open garden two to four weeks before frost-free date. Keep soil evenly moist with mulch throughout growing season. When plants are six weeks old, sidedress with well-composted manure or manure tea.

Harvest and Storage: Dig roots before ground freezes, (generally 65 to 150 days after seeds are sown) and trim away all but 1 inch of leaves. Replant roots indoors in 10 inches of moist soil, topped off by 6 to 8 inches of sterilized, dampened sand or sawdust. When blanched chicons show through top layer (in about three weeks), they are ready to harvest for salads. Separate chicons where they join roots.

Appendix

The Best of the Garden on the Dinner Table:
A Year-Round Guide to Balanced Nutrition

Nutrient	In Spring	In Summer	In Autumn	In Winter*

Protein	Dry beans
	Peas**
		Cowpeas**
		Lima
		  beans**
			Peanuts
			Sunflower
			  seeds
				Dry beans
				Sunflower
				  seeds

Calcium	Dandelion
	  greens**
	Spinach**
	Leaf
	  lettuce**
		Amaranth**
		Collards**
		Turnip
		  greens**
		Broccoli**
		Okra**
		Kale**
			Amaranth**
			Collards**
			Broccoli**
				Frozen
				  vege-
				  tables
				Almonds

Phosphorus	Nuts
	Dry beans
		Cowpeas**
		Broccoli**
		Lima
		  beans**
			Sunflower
			  seeds
			Nuts
			Broccoli**
				Nuts
				Dry beans

Iron	Straw-
	  berries**
	Butterhead
	  lettuce**
	Spinach**
	Peas**
		Amaranth**
		Lima
		  beans**
		Water-
		  melons**
		Cowpeas**
			Dry beans
			Frozen
			  lima beans
			Fall
			  spinach**
				Dry beans
				Frozen
				  vege-
				  tables

Potassium	Dry beans
	Lettuce**
		Potatoes**
		Amaranth**
		Water-
		  melons**
		New
		  Zealand
		  spinach**
		Broccoli**
			Potatoes**
			Winter
			  squash**
			Broccoli**
				Potatoes
				Winter
				  squash
				Dry beans

*In winter, use potatoes, winter squash, sweet potatoes, onions, and turnips from the root cellar. During fall and winter, fill in nutritional gaps with frozen or canned vegetables and fruits.

**Fresh from the garden.

Nutrient	In Spring	In Summer	In Autumn	In Winter*
Vitamin A	Dandelion greens** Spinach** Garden cress**	Carrots** Collards** Amaranth** Chard**	Sweet potatoes** Carrots** Collards** Winter squash	Sweet potatoes Winter squash
Thiamine	Peas** Dandelion greens**	Cowpeas** Lima beans** Okra** Potatoes**	Onions** Potatoes**	Dry beans Onions Potatoes
Riboflavin	Dandelion greens** Spinach**	Broccoli** Okra** Amaranth** Collards**	Winter squash** Broccoli** Collards**	Mushrooms Winter squash
Niacin	Potatoes Mushrooms Peas**	Potatoes** Amaranth** Cowpeas**	Peanuts Potatoes** Sunflower seeds	Potatoes Mushrooms Sunflower seeds
Vitamin C	Strawberries** Spinach** Peas**	Broccoli** Amaranth** Sweet peppers** Brussels sprouts** Collards** Cabbage** Kohlrabi**	Broccoli** Brussels sprouts** Collards** Cabbage** Kohlrabi**	Potatoes Sweet potatoes Turnips

Nutrient Content of Fruits and Vegetables

Food	Serving Portion	Calories	Protein (g)	Calcium (mg)	Phosphorus (mg)
Almonds	¼ cup, raw, shelled	194	6.1	83	164
Amaranth	4 oz., raw	41	4.0	303	76
Apples	1 med., 5⅓ oz., raw	80	0.3	10	14
Apricots	3 fruits, 4 oz., raw	55	1.1	18	25
Asparagus	4 med. spears, 2 oz., cooked	12	1.3	13	30
Avocados	½ med., raw	188	2.4	11	47
Beans, great northern	½ cup, cooked	106	7.0	45	133
Beans, green snap	½ cup, cooked	16	1.0	32	23
Beans, kidney	½ cup, cooked	114	7.2	45	130
Beans, lima	½ cup, cooked	95	6.5	40	103
Beans, navy	½ cup, cooked	112	7.4	48	141
Beans, yellow wax	½ cup, cooked	14	0.9	32	23
Beet greens	½ cup, cooked	13	1.3	72	18
Beet roots	½ cup, cooked, diced	27	1.0	12	20
Blackberries	½ cup, raw	42	0.9	23	14
Blueberries	½ cup, raw	45	0.5	11	10
Broccoli	5-oz. stalk, cooked	36	4.3	123	87

SOURCE: *U.S. Department of Agriculture, Agriculture Handbook No. 456, Nutritive Value of American Foods in Common Units.*

Iron (mg)	Sodium (mg)	Potassium (mg)	Vitamin A (I.U.)	Thiamine (mg)	Riboflavin (mg)	Niacin (mg)	Vitamin C (mg)
1.5	1.5	275	0	0.09	0.33	1.3	trace
4.4	—	466	6,918	0.09	0.18	1.6	91
0.4	1.0	152	120	0.04	0.03	0.1	6*
0.5	1.0	301	2,890	0.03	0.04	0.6	11
0.4	1.0	110	540	0.10	0.11	0.8	16
0.7	5.0	680	330	0.12	0.23	1.8	16
2.5	6.5	375	0	0.13	0.07	0.7	0
0.4	2.5	95	340	0.04	0.05	0.2	7
2.2	3.0	315	5	0.10	0.06	0.7	—
2.2	1.0	359	240	240	0.16	0.09	1.1
2.6	6.5	395	0	0.14	0.07	0.7	0
0.4	2.0	95	145	0.05	0.06	0.3	8
1.4	55.0	241	3,700	0.05	0.11	0.2	11
0.5	37.0	177	15	0.03	0.04	0.3	5
0.7	0.5	123	145	0.02	0.03	0.3	15
0.8	0.5	59	75	0.02	0.05	0.4	10
1.1	14.0	374	3,500	0.13	0.28	1.1	126

*See discussion of high-vitamin varieties in the box, Superior Apple Varieties in chapter 2.

(continued)

Nutrient Content of Fruits and Vegetables—*continued*

Food	Serving Portion	Calories	Protein (g)	Calcium (mg)	Phosphorus (mg)
Brussels sprouts	½ cup, cooked (4 sprouts)	28	3.3	25	56
Cabbage	1 cup, raw, chopped	22	1.2	44	26
Carrots	1 med., 2⅞ oz., raw	30	0.8	27	26
Cauliflower	½ cup, cooked	14	1.5	13	27
Celery	8-in. stalk, 1½ oz., raw	7	0.4	16	11
Chard	½ cup, cooked	16	1.6	64	21
Cherries, sour	½ cup, 4 oz., raw	30	0.6	12	10
Cherries, sweet	½ cup, 4 oz., raw	41	0.8	13	11
Chinese cabbage	½ cup, 2½ oz., raw, chopped	6	0.5	16	15
Collards	½ cup, cooked	30	3.3	168	46
Corn	½ cup, cooked	69	2.7	3	74
Cowpeas	½ cup, cooked	89	6.7	20	121
Cucumbers	½ cup, 1⅞ oz., sliced	8	0.5	13	14
Dandelion greens	½ cup, 3¾ oz., cooked	35	2.1	147	44
Eggplants	½ cup, cooked, diced	47	1.0	11	21
Endive	1 cup, 1¾ oz., raw, chopped	10	0.9	41	27
Garden cress	½ cup, cooked	15	1.2	39	30
Globe artichokes	1 med., 10½ oz., cooked	10–53**	3.4	61	83
Gooseberries	½ cup, raw	30	0.6	14	12

**Least when freshly harvested; calories increase with storage time.

Iron (mg)	Sodium (mg)	Potassium (mg)	Vitamin A (I.U.)	Thiamine (mg)	Riboflavin (mg)	Niacin (mg)	Vitamin C (mg)
0.9	8.0	212	405	0.06	0.11	0.6	68
0.4	18	210	120	0.05	0.05	0.3	42
0.5	34.0	246	7,930	0.04	0.04	0.4	6
0.5	5.5	129	40	0.06	0.05	0.4	35
0.1	50.0	136	110	0.01	0.01	0.1	4
1.6	76.0	281	4,725	0.04	0.10	0.4	14
0.2	1.0	98	515	0.03	0.03	0.2	5
0.3	1.0	112	65	0.03	0.04	0.3	6
0.3	9.0	95	55	0.02	0.02	0.3	10
0.8	—	231	7,410	0.07	0.14	1.1	49
0.5	trace	136	330	0.09	0.09	1.1	6
1.8	1.0	313	290	0.25	0.09	1.2	14
0.6	3.0	84	130	0.02	0.02	0.1	6
1.9	46.0	244	12,290	0.14	0.17	—	19
0.6	1.0	150	10	0.05	0.04	0.5	3
0.9	7.0	147	1,650	0.04	0.07	0.3	5
0.5	5.5	222	4,725	0.03	0.10	0.5	16
1.3	36.0	361	180	0.08	0.05	0.8	10
0.4	2.0	117	220	—	—	—	25

(continued)

Nutrient Content of Fruits and Vegetables—*continued*

Food	Serving Portion	Calories	Protein (g)	Calcium (mg)	Phosphorus (mg)
Grapefruit	½ med., 3⁹⁄₁₆-in. diameter	40	0.5	16	16
Grapes, Concord	10 grapes, 1½ oz.	18	0.3	4	3
Honeydew melons	7 by 2-in. wedge, 8 oz.	49	1.2	21	24
Kale	½ cup, cooked	22	2.5	103	32
Kohlrabi	½ cup, cooked, diced	20	1.4	27	34
Lemons	½ fruit, 2¼-in. diameter	12	0.5	12	7
Lentils	½ cup, cooked	106	7.8	25	119
Lettuce, butterhead	4 oz., raw	16	1.4	40	30
Lettuce, iceberg	4 oz., raw	15	1.0	23	25
Lettuce, leaf	4 oz., raw	21	1.5	77	28
Lettuce, romaine	4 oz., raw	21	1.5	77	28
Loganberries	½ cup, raw	45	0.7	25	12
Mushrooms	2 oz., raw	16	1.5	3	66
Muskmelons	¼ fruit, 5-in. diameter, 8½ oz.	41	1.0	19	22
Mustard greens	½ cup, cooked	16	1.6	97	23
New Zealand spinach	½ cup, cooked	12	1.6	43	25
Okra	4 oz., cooked	33	2.3	104	47
Onions, dry	2 oz., raw	22	0.9	15	20
Onions, green	2 oz., raw	20	0.9	29	22
Oranges	1 med., 2⅝-in. diameter	64	1.3	54	26
Peaches	1 med., 2¾-in. diameter	58	0.9	14	29

Iron (mg)	Sodium (mg)	Potassium (mg)	Vitamin A (I.U.)	Thiamine (mg)	Riboflavin (mg)	Niacin (mg)	Vitamin C (mg)
0.4	1.0	132	80	0.04	0.02	0.2	37
0.1	1.0	42	30	0.01	0.01	0.1	1
0.6	18.0	374	60	0.06	0.04	0.9	34
0.9	24.0	122	4,565	0.05	0.10	0.9	51
0.3	5.0	215	15	0.05	0.03	0.2	36
0.3	1.0	60	10	0.02	0.01	0.1	23
2.1	—	249	20	0.07	0.06	0.6	0
2.3	10.3	300	1,100	0.07	0.07	0.4	9
0.6	10.3	199	375	0.07	0.07	0.4	7
1.6	10.3	300	2,155	0.06	0.09	0.5	21
1.6	10.3	300	2,155	0.06	0.09	0.5	21
0.9	0.5	123	145	0.02	0.03	0.3	18
0.5	8.5	235	trace	0.06	0.26	2.4	2
0.6	16.5	341	4,620	0.06	0.04	0.8	45
1.3	12.5	154	4,060	0.06	0.10	0.4	34
1.4	83.0	417	3,240	0.03	0.09	0.5	13
0.6	2.3	197	555	0.15	0.21	1.0	23
0.3	5.6	89	23	0.18	0.02	0.1	6
0.6	2.9	131	1,134	0.03	0.03	0.2	18
0.5	1.0	263	260	0.13	0.05	0.5	66
0.8	2.0	308	2,030	0.03	0.08	1.5	11

(continued)

Nutrient Content of Fruits and Vegetables—*continued*

Food	Serving Portion	Calories	Protein (g)	Calcium (mg)	Phosphorus (mg)
Peanuts	¼ cup, roasted, shelled	210	9.4	26	147
Pears	1 med., 2½ by 3½ in., raw	100	1.1	13	18
Peas	½ cup, cooked	57	4.3	19	79
Pecans	¼ cup, roasted, shelled	186	2.5	20	78
Peppers, sweet	2½-oz. fruit, raw	13	0.7	6	13
Plums	5 med., 1-in. diameter	33	0.3	9	9
Popcorn	3 cups, popped, ⅔ oz.	69	2.4	3	51
Potatoes	1 med., 7⅛ oz., baked	145	4.0	14	101
Radishes	5 radishes, ¾–1-in. diameter	4	0.3	7	7
Raspberries, black	½ cup, raw	49	1.0	20	15
Raspberries, red	½ cup, raw	35	0.8	14	14
Rhubarb	½ cup, 2¼ oz., raw, diced	10	0.4	59	11
Rutabagas	½ cup, cooked, mashed	42	1.1	71	37
Salsify	½ cup, cooked, cubed	8–47**	1.8	29	36
Soybeans	½ cup, cooked	117	9.9	66	161
Spinach	1 cup, 2 oz., raw, chopped	14	1.8	51	28
Spinach	½ cup, 3⅛ oz., cooked	21	2.7	84	34
Squash, acorn	½ cup, baked, mashed	57	2.0	40	30

Iron (mg)	Sodium (mg)	Potassium (mg)	Vitamin A (I.U.)	Thiamine (mg)	Riboflavin (mg)	Niacin (mg)	Vitamin C (mg)
0.8	1.8	252	—	0.12	0.05	6.2	0
0.5	3.0	213	30	0.03	0.07	0.2	7
1.5	1.0	157	430	0.23	0.09	1.9	32
0.7	trace	163	35	0.23	0.04	0.3	1
0.4	8.0	124	244	0.05	0.05	0.3	74
0.3	1.0	150	150	0.04	0.02	0.3	—
0.6	trace	—	—	—	0.03	0.3	0
1.1	6.0	782	trace	0.15	0.07	2.7	31
0.3	4.0	73	trace	0.01	0.01	0.1	6
0.6	0.5	134	trace	0.02	0.06	0.06	12
0.6	0.5	104	80	0.02	0.06	0.6	16
0.5	1.0	153	60	0.02	0.05	0.2	6
0.4	5.0	201	660	0.07	0.07	1.0	31
0.9	—	180	5	0.02	0.03	0.2	5
2.5	2.0	486	25	0.19	0.08	0.6	0
1.7	39.0	259	4,460	0.06	0.11	0.3	28
2.0	45.0	292	7,290	0.07	0.13	0.5	25
1.2	1.0	492	1,435	0.05	0.14	0.7	14

(continued)

Nutrient Content of Fruits and Vegetables—*continued*

Food	Serving Portion	Calories	Protein (g)	Calcium (mg)	Phosphorus (mg)
Squash, butternut	½ cup, baked, mashed	70	1.9	41	74
Squash, crookneck	½ cup, boiled, mashed	18	1.2	30	30
Squash, Hubbard	½ cup, baked, mashed	52	1.9	25	40
Squash, scallop	½ cup, boiled, mashed	19	0.9	30	30
Squash, zucchini	½ cup, boiled, mashed	15	1.2	30	30
Strawberries	½ cup, 2⅝ oz., whole berries	28	0.5	16	16
Sunflower seeds	¼ cup, raw, hulled	203	8.7	44	304
Sweet potatoes	1 med., 5⅛ oz., baked	161	2.4	46	66
Tomatoes	1 med., 4¾ oz., raw	27	1.4	16	33
Turnip greens	½ cup, cooked	14	1.6	126	25
Turnip roots	½ cup, cooked, mashed	27	0.9	41	28
Walnuts, black	1 oz., shelled	178	5.8	trace	162
Walnuts, English	1 oz., shelled	185	4.2	28	108
Watercress	10 sprigs, 1¼ oz.	7	0.8	53	19
Watermelons	1-in.-thick, 10-in.-diameter slice	111	2.1	30	43
Witloof chicory	½ cup, 3¼ oz., chopped	7	0.5	8	10

Iron (mg)	Sodium (mg)	Potassium (mg)	Vitamin A (I.U.)	Thiamine (mg)	Riboflavin (mg)	Niacin (mg)	Vitamin C (mg)
1.1	1.0	624	6,560	0.05	0.14	0.7	8
0.5	1.0	169	530	0.06	0.10	1.0	13
0.8	1.0	278	4,920	0.05	0.14	0.7	11
0.5	1.0	169	215	0.06	0.10	1.0	10
0.5	1.0	169	360	0.06	0.10	1.0	11
0.8	1.0	122	45	0.02	0.05	0.5	44
2.6	11.0	334	18	0.71	0.08	2.0	—
1.0	14.0	342	9,230	0.10	0.08	0.8	25
0.6	4.0	300	1,100	0.07	0.05	0.9	28
0.8	—	—	4,135	0.08	0.17	0.4	34
0.5	39.0	216	trace	0.05	0.06	0.4	26
1.7	1.0	130	90	0.06	0.03	0.2	—
0.9	1.0	128	10	0.09	0.04	0.3	1
0.6	18.0	99	1,720	0.03	0.06	0.3	28
2.1	4.0	426	2,510	0.13	0.13	0.9	30
0.3	3.0	82	trace	—	—	—	—

Seed Sources for Superior Vegetables and Fruits

Amaranth (listed under a variety of names in various seed catalogs)
  Burpee (tampala)
  Dr. Yoo Farm (Chinese spinach)
  Grace's Garden (hin choy)
  Nichols Garden Nursery (edible amaranth spinach)
  Park Seed (tampala)
  Redwood City (amaranth)
  Tsang and Ma International (hin choy)

Adzuki Beans
  Thompson and Morgan
  Vermont Bean Seed

Apple Varieties (The varieties listed in chapter 2 are widely available; given here are major mail-order nurseries.)
  Burgess
  Burpee
  Earl May
  Farmer
  Gurney
  Henry Field
  Kelly Brothers
  Redwood City

Imperator Carrots
  Burpee
  Farmer
  Henry Field

Early Snowball Cauliflower
  Burgess
  Earl May
  Gurney
  Herbst Brothers
  Stokes
  Thompson and Morgan

Dwarf Scotch Kale
  Burgess
  Farmer
  Gurney
  Johnny's Selected Seeds
  Stokes

Soybeans
  Burpee
  Earl May
  Farmer
  Gurney
  Vermont Bean Seed

Eat-All Squash (also listed as Sweet Nut squash)
  Farmer

Jersey Golden Acorn Squash
  Burpee
  Park Seed

Kuta Squash
  Park Seed

Mammoth Russian Sunflowers
  Stokes

Allgold Sweet Potatoes
  Farmer
  Gurney
  Henry Field
  Park Seed

Centennial Sweet Potatoes
  Earl May
  Gurney
  Henry Field

Georgia Red Sweet Potatoes
  Park Seed

Porto Rico Sweet Potatoes
Earl May
Gurney
Henry Field

Caro-Red Tomatoes
Burgess
Farmer
Gurney
Stokes
Thompson and Morgan

Caro-Rich Tomatoes
Burgess

Doublerich Tomatoes
Burgess
Farmer
Shumway

Charleston Gray Watermelons
Burgess
Burpee
Gurney
Henry Field
Herbst Brothers

Seed Sources Directory

Burgess Seed and Plant Co.
905 Four Seasons Rd.
Bloomington, IL 61701

W. Atlee Burpee Co.
Burpee Bldg.
Warminster, PA 18974

Dr. Yoo Farm
Box 290
College Park, MD 20740

Earl May Seed and Nursery Co.
100 N. Elm
Shenandoah, IA 51603

Farmer Seed and Nursery Co.
818 N.W. Fourth St.
Faribault, MN 55021

Grace's Garden
10 Bay St.
Westport, CT 06880

Gurney Seed and Nursery Co.
Yankton, SD 57079

Henry Field Seed and Nursery
407 Sycamore
Shenandoah, IA 51602

Herbst Brothers Seedsmen, Inc.
1000 N. Main St.
Brewster, NY 10509

Johnny's Selected Seeds
Albion, ME 04910

Kelly Brothers Nurseries
Dansville, NY 14437

Nichols Garden Nursery
1190 North Pacific Highway
Albany, OR 97321

George W. Park Seed Co.
Box 31
Greenwood, SC 29647

Redwood City Seed Co.
P.O. Box 361
Redwood City, CA 94064

R. H. Shumway Seedsman, Inc.
628 Cedar St.
Rockford, IL 61101

Stokes Seeds, Inc.
P.O. Box 548
737 Main St.
Buffalo, NY 14240

Thompson and Morgan, Inc.
P.O. Box 100
Farmingdale, NJ 07727

Vermont Bean Seed Company
Garden Ln.
Bomoseen, VT 05732

Tsang and Ma International
1306 Old Country Rd.
Belmont, CA 94002

Notes

Chapter 1

1. *Food Consumption, Prices and Expenditures,* Statistical Bulletin No. 138, and succeeding supplements, Economic Research Service, United States Department of Agriculture.

2. M. Allen Stevens, "Varietal Influence on Nutritional Value," *Nutritional Qualities of Fresh Fruits and Vegetables,* ed. Philip L. White (Mount Kisco, N.Y.: Futura Publishing Co., 1974), pp. 87–108.

Chapter 2

1. Edwin A. Crosby, "The Economics of Genetic Engineering," *Nutritional Qualities of Fresh Fruits and Vegetables,* ed. Philip L. White (Mount Kisco, N.Y.: Futura Publishing Co., 1974), pp. 169–75.

2. Ross Hume Hall, "The Agri-Business View of Soil and Life," *Journal of Holistic Medicine,* 3:2 (Human Sciences Press, Fall/Winter, 1981), p. 157.

3. C. C. Strachen et al., *Chemical Composition and Nutritive Value of British Columbia Tree Fruits,* Publication No. 862, Canada Department of Agriculture, 1951.

4. T. P. Hernandez et al., "Inheritance of and Method of Rating Flesh Color in *Ipomoea batatas,*" *Proceedings of the American Society of Horticultural Science,* vol. 87 (1965), pp. 387–90.

5. M. L. Tormes et al., "The Carotene Pigment Content of Certain Red Fleshed Watermelons," *Proceedings of the American Society for Horticultural Science,* vol. 82 (1963), pp. 460–64.

Chapter 3

1. M. Allby and F. Allen, *Robots Behind the Plow* (Emmaus, Pa.: Rodale Press, 1974), p. 19.

2. Walter Ebeling, "The Relation of Soil Quality to the Nutritional Value of Plant Crops," *Journal of Applied Nutrition,* 33:1 (1981), p. 20.

3. W. P. Bitters, "Physical Characteristics and Chemical Composition as Affected by Scions and Rootstocks," *The Orange,* ed. W. B. Sinclair (University of California Division of Agricultural Sciences, 1961), pp. 56–95.

4. O. Sheets, *The Relationship of Soil Fertility to Human Nutrition,* Mississippi Agricultural Experiment Station Bulletin No. 437, 1946.

5. K. C. Hammer et al., "Effects of Light Intensity, Day Length, Temperature, and Other Environmental Factors on the Ascorbic Acid Content of Tomatoes," *Journal of Nutrition,* 29 (1944), pp. 85–97.

6. Walter Ebeling, "How Fertilizers Affect the Nutrient Balance in Plant Crops," *Journal of Applied Nutrition,* 33:2 (1981), pp. 138–55.

7. S. L. Tisdale and W. L. Nelson, *Soil Fertility and Fertilizers* (New York: Macmillan, 1966).

8. Walter Ebeling, "How Fertilizers Affect Nutrient Balance," pp. 138–55.

9. Dietrich Knorr, *Food Science and Technology,* 12 (1979), pp. 350–56.

10. Walter Ebeling, "How Fertilizers Affect Nutrient Balance," pp. 138–39.

11. R. McCarrison, *Indian Journal of Medical Research,* 14, p. 351.

12. W. Schuphan, *Ernahrungs-Umschau,* 21 (1974), p. 103.

13. Dietrich Knorr, *Food Science and Technology,* 12 (1979), pp. 350–56.

14. W. Schuphan, *Mensch und Nahrungspflanze,* Dr. W. Junk. B. V. Verlag, Den Haag, 1976.

15. P. Handler, *Metabolism* (Federation of American Societies for Experimental Biology, 1965).

16. Dietrich Knorr, *Food Science and Technology,* 12 (1979), pp. 350–56.

Chapter 4

1. M. Allen Stevens, "Varietal Influence on Nutritional Value," *Nutritional Qualities of Fresh Fruits and Vegetables,* ed. Philip L. White (Mount Kisco, N.Y.: Futura Publishing Co., 1974), p. 90.

Chapter 6

1. G. Fred Somers and Kenneth C. Beeson, *Advances in Food Research,* vol. 1 (1948), pp. 299–300.

2. Robert S. Harris and Harry Von Loesecke, *Nutritional Evaluation of Food Processing* (New York: John Wiley and Sons, 1960), pp. 58–86, 418–35, 462–82.

3. E. E. C. Fager et al., "Folic Acid in Vegetables and Certain Other Plant Materials," *Food Research,* 14 (1949), pp. 1–8.

4. L. P. Pepkowitz, "The Carotene and Ascorbic Acid Concentration of Vegetable Varieties," *Plant Physiology,* 19 (1944), pp. 615–26.

5. W. C. Dietrich et al. "The Time-Temperature Tolerance of Frozen Foods," *Food Technology* (1957), pp. 109–13.

6. Anthony DeCrosta, "Save Those Vitamins!" *Organic Gardening* (August, 1979), p. 81.

7. R. E. Hein and I. J. Hutchings, "Influence of Processing on Vitamin-Mineral Content and Biological Availability in Processed Foods," symposium report, American Medical Association Council on Foods and Nutrition, 1971.

8. Ibid.

9. H. O. Werner and R. M. Leverton, "The Ascorbic Acid Content of Nebraska-grown Potatoes as Influenced by Variety, Environment, Maturity and Storage," *American Potato Journal*, 23 (1946), pp. 265–67.

10. S. V. Bring and F. P. Raab, "Total Ascorbic Acid in Potatoes," *Journal of the American Dietetic Association*, 45 (1964) pp. 149–52.

11. Harris and Von Loesecke, *Nutritional Evaluation* (1960), pp. 58–86, 418–35, 462–82.

12. C. Y. Lee et al., "The Variations of Ascorbic Acid Content in Vegetable Processing," *Journal of Food Chemistry*, 1 (1976), p. 15.

13. Harris and Von Loesecke, *Nutritional Evaluation* (1960), pp. 58–86, 418–35, 462–82.

14. Godavari Kamalanathan et al., "The Effect of Boiling, Steaming, Pressure Cooking and Panning on the Mineral and Vitamin Content of Three Vegetables," *Indian Journal of Nutrition and Dietetics*, 11:10 (1974), p. 19.

15. E. M. Hewston et al., *Vitamin and Mineral Content of Certain Foods as Affected by Home Preparation*, United States Department of Agriculture Misc. Pub. No. 628.

Recommended Reading

Stoner, Carol H. and the Editors of *Organic Gardening and Farming* Magazine. *Stocking Up*. rev. ed. Emmaus, Pa.: Rodale Press, 1977.

Editors of *Organic Gardening* Magazine. *Getting the Most from Your Garden*. Emmaus, Pa.: Rodale Press, 1980.

Editors of Rodale Press. *The Organic Gardener's Complete Guide to Vegetables and Fruits*. Emmaus, Pa.: Rodale Press, 1982.

Faelten, Sharon and the Editors of *Prevention* Magazine. *The Complete Book of Minerals for Health*. rev. ed. Emmaus, Pa.: Rodale Press, 1981.

Lappé, Frances Moore. *Diet for a Small Planet*, rev. ed. New York: Ballantine Books, 1975.

Newcomb, Duane. *Growing Vegetables the Big Yield/Small Space Way*. Los Angeles: J. P. Tarcher, 1981.

Staff of *Prevention* Magazine. *The Complete Book of Vitamins*. Emmaus, Pa.: Rodale Press, 1977.

Sussman, Vic. *The Vegetarian Alternative*. Emmaus, Pa.: Rodale Press, 1978.

Index

Page numbers in boldface indicate table entries and boxed material.